The Retina
in Systemic Disease

A Color Manual
of Ophthalmoscopy

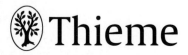

The Retina in Systemic Disease

A Color Manual of Ophthalmoscopy

Homayoun Tabandeh, MD, MS, FRCP, FRCS, FRCOphth
Retina-Vitreous Associates
Los Angeles, California
Former Director, Retina Service
Department of Ophthalmology
University of Florida
Gainesville, Florida

Morton F. Goldberg, MD, FACS, FAOS, Dr.hon.causa
Joseph E. Green Professor of Ophthalmology
Former Director, The Wilmer Eye Institute
Johns Hopkins University School of Medicine
Baltimore, Maryland

Thieme
New York • Stuttgart

Thieme Medical Publishers, Inc.
333 Seventh Ave.
New York, NY 10001

Editorial Director: Michael Wachinger
Managing Editor: J. Owen Zurhellen IV
Editorial Assistant: Dominik Pucek
Vice President, Production and Electronic Publishing: Anne T. Vinnicombe
Production Editor: Kenneth L. Chumbley, Publication Services
Vice President, International Marketing and Sales: Cornelia Schulze
Chief Financial Officer: Peter van Woerden
President: Brian D. Scanlan
Compositor: MPS Content Services, A Macmillan Company
Printer: Gobsons Papers Ltd.

Library of Congress Cataloging-in-Publication Data

Tabandeh, Homayoun.
  The Retina in Systemic Disease: A Color Manual of Ophthalmoscopy / Homayoun Tabandeh, Morton F. Goldberg.
    p. ; cm.
  Includes index.
  ISBN 978-1-60406-055-3 (alk. paper)
  1. Retina—Examination—Atlases 2. Ocular manifestations of general diseases—Atlases. 3. Ophthalmoscopy—Atlases. I. Goldberg, Morton F. II. Title.
  [DNLM: 1. Retina—pathology—Atlases. 2. Diagnosis, Differential—Atlases. 3. Eye Manifestations—Atlases. 4. Ophthalmoscopy—methods—Atlases.
WW 17 T112c 2009]
  RE551.T33 2009
  617.7'350222—dc22

                                                                  2008045198

Important note: Medical knowledge is ever-changing. As new research and clinical experience broaden our knowledge, changes in treatment and drug therapy may be required. The authors and editors of the material herein have consulted sources believed to be reliable in their efforts to provide information that is complete and in accord with the standards accepted at the time of publication. However, in view of the possibility of human error by the authors, editors, or publisher of the work herein or changes in medical knowledge, neither the authors, editors, nor publisher, nor any other party who has been involved in the preparation of this work, warrants that the information contained herein is in every respect accurate or complete, and they are not responsible for any errors or omissions or for the results obtained from use of such information. Readers are encouraged to confirm the information contained herein with other sources. For example, readers are advised to check the product information sheet included in the package of each drug they plan to administer to be certain that the information contained in this publication is accurate and that changes have not been made in the recommended dose or in the contraindications for administration. This recommendation is of particular importance in connection with new or infrequently used drugs.

Some of the product names, patents, and registered designs referred to in this book are in fact registered trademarks or proprietary names even though specific reference to this fact is not always made in the text. Therefore, the appearance of a name without designation as proprietary is not to be construed as a representation by the publisher that it is in the public domain.

Printed in India

5 4 3 2 1

ISBN 978-1-60406-055-3

To my family, teachers, and students.

Homayoun Tabandeh

To Myrna D. Goldberg, MSW, Matthew F. Goldberg, JD,
and Michael F. Goldberg, MD, MPH.

Morton F. Goldberg

Contents

Foreword

One of my children's favorite bedtime stories was about an old man from a village who dreamt of a fabulous treasure buried in a distant land. Only after trekking through forests, sailing across seas, and climbing mountains did the old man learn that the treasure he had dreamt of was actually hidden under the stove of his house back in the village! In medical diagnosis, as in fables, treasures are often buried right under our nose. Examination of the retina affords an unparalleled opportunity for the physician to diagnose at the bedside a systemic disease and to save the patient from having to trek through forests of laboratory tests or swim past a sea of consultants. Ophthalmoscopy also frequently permits physicians to judge the activity or severity of many diseases, from the common (e.g., diabetes, hypertension) to the unusual (e.g., vasculitis, sarcoidosis). Unfortunately, many physicians do not—metaphorically—move the stove in their own kitchen (i.e., grab their ophthalmoscopes).

Fortunately, this book will help any physician learn or reclaim the art of examining the retina for signs of systemic diseases. Simple and clear instructions on how to position the patient and the examiner, how to hold the ophthalmoscope, and how to dilate the eyes will help physicians overcome some of the obstacles to an effective examination. The liberal use of bulleted summary points makes this manual both concise and thorough. Physicians from neurosurgeons to rheumatologists to general internists and family physicians will enjoy the high quality photographs that illustrate important retinal findings relevant to these different disciplines.

I wish that this color manual of the retina had been available to me when I was training in internal medicine and rheumatology. I believe this book will allow many physicians to experience the joy of using ophthalmoscopy to quickly discover the many diagnostic treasures of systemic disorders present in the retinas of their patients.

David B. Hellmann, MD, MACP
Aliki Perroti Professor of Medicine
Vice Dean, Johns Hopkins Bayview Medical Center
Chairman, Department of Medicine Johns Hopkins Bayview
The Johns Hopkins University School of Medicine
Baltimore, Maryland

Preface

Examination of the human retina provides an excellent and unique opportunity for the direct study of nervous, vascular, and connective tissues. Many systemic disorders have retinal manifestations that are valuable in screening, diagnosis, staging, or management of these conditions. Retinal involvement in systemic disorders, such as diabetes mellitus, is a major cause of morbidity and impairment of quality of life. Early recognition by screening is a key factor in effective treatment.

Ophthalmoscopy has the potential to be one of the most "high yield" aspects of physical examination performed by physicians of any specialty. In spite of its tremendous value, most physicians feel uncomfortable performing ophthalmoscopy and wish for better training and for access to a convenient source of authoritative and focused information on the subject. Challenges occur at multiple levels, including the practical aspects of performing ophthalmoscopy, recognition and understanding of retinal findings in systemic disease, and their differential diagnosis.

The aim of this book is to provide an illustrated manual of the basic principles and practical aspects of ophthalmoscopy. Concise and clear descriptions of retinal signs and their differential diagnosis and retinal manifestations of systemic disease are provided. Numerous high-quality color clinical photographs illustrate each topic. Treatment of retinal conditions has not been covered in order to keep the focus firmly on the recognition and diagnosis of abnormal fundus findings.

The first section deals with the basic and practical aspects of ophthalmoscopy. The second section illustrates various retinal signs and lists the differential diagnosis. The third section covers the retinal manifestations of a wide range of systemic disorders.

The authors hope that this book serves as a useful and enjoyable pictorial reference for medical students, ophthalmologists, optometrists, and physicians of many specialties.

Acknowledgments

The authors wish to thank the following physicians who kindly contributed clinical photographs to be included in this manual: David S. Boyer, Neil Bressler, Susan Bressler, Margaret Chang, Thomas G. Chu, Diana Do, James P. Dunn, Charles Eberhardt, Geoffrey Emerson, Michael Emerson, Christina Flaxel, Daniel Garibaldi, W. Richard Green, James Handa, J. Jill Hopkins, Peter J. McDonnell, Neil R. Miller, Timothy G. Murray, Quan Nguyen, Roger L. Novack, Cameron F. Parsa, Nastaran Rafiei, Firas M. Rahhal, Michael X. Repka, Vivian Rismondo, Richard Roe, Steven D. Schwartz, Edgar L. Thomas, and Elias Traboulsi.

The authors also wish to thank the following individuals for their assistance: Pinoi Bouddhabandith, Tony Dyrek, Don Enkerud, Cathie Felter, Stacey Halper, Hector Jimenez, Jeff Kessinger, Eric Protacio, Julio Sierra, Dean Smith, Adam Smucker, Amir Saidi (art consultant), Massoud Saidi, and Trina Toyama. Finally, the authors wish to thank the following departments and institutes for their assistance: the Department of Photography at the Retina-Vitreous Associates Medical Group, Los Angeles, California; the Wilmer Eye Institute, Baltimore, Maryland; and the Department of Ophthalmology of the University of Florida, Gainesville, Florida.

Examination of the Retina

1 Anatomy of the Eye

The eye consists of a shell (cornea and sclera), crystalline lens, iris diaphragm, ciliary body, choroid, and the retina. Aqueous humor fills the space between the cornea and the lens (anterior chamber). The space between the posterior aspect of the lens and retina is filled by vitreous. The choroid and the retina cover the posterior two thirds of the sclera internally (**Fig. 1.1**).

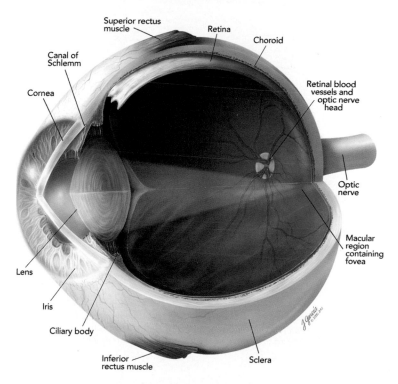

Fig. 1.1 Structure of the eye—section of the left eye showing the internal and external structures. The fovea is situated 2.5 disc diameters (approximately 4.5 mm) temporal to the optic disc. (Drawing by Juan R. Garcia. Used with permission from Johns Hopkins University.)

The choroid is located between the sclera and the retina, and consists of three layers:

◆ Outer layer—large vessels
◆ Middle layer—medium-size vessels
◆ Inner layer—choriocapillary layer

Bruch's membrane is a specialized basement membrane that separates the choriocapillary layer from the overlying retinal pigment epithelium (RPE) layer. It is derived from the basement membrane of the choriocapillaries and the RPE. The RPE layer is adherent to the overlying retinal photoreceptor cells by specialized cellular interdigitations and by an active cellular pump mechanism (**Fig. 1.2**).

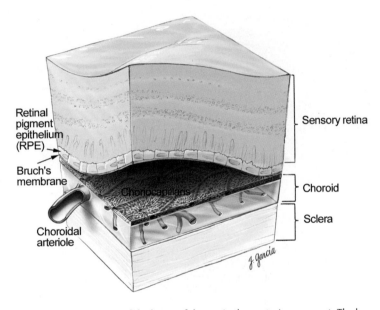

Fig. 1.2 Cross section of the layers of the eye in the posterior segment. The layers include neurosensory retina, retinal pigment epithelium, Bruch's membrane, choroid, and sclera. (Drawing by Juan R. Garcia. Used with permission from Johns Hopkins University.)

The retina consists of various layers of specialized cells, including photoreceptors, bipolar cells, amacrine cells, Müller cells, and ganglion cells (**Fig. 1.3**).

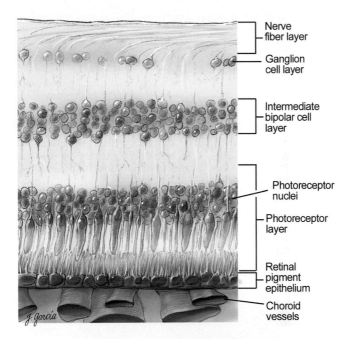

Nerve fiber layer

Ganglion cell layer

Intermediate bipolar cell layer

Photoreceptor nuclei

Photoreceptor layer

Retinal pigment epithelium

Choroid vessels

Fig. 1.3 Cross-sectional diagram of the retinal layers. The layers of the retina and choroid, from innermost outward, are as follows: 1, internal limiting membrane; 2, nerve fiber layer; 3, ganglion cell layer; 4, inner plexiform layer; 5, inner nuclear layer; 6, outer plexiform layer; 7, outer nuclear layer; 8, photoreceptor outer segment layer; 9, retinal pigment epithelium; 10, Bruch's membrane; 11, choroid. (Drawing by Juan R. Garcia. Used with permission from Johns Hopkins University.)

◆ The Macula

The macula is the central part of the retina, and is responsible for detailed vision (acuity) and color perception. The macula is defined clinically as the area of the retina centered on the posterior pole of the fundus, measuring approximately 5 disc diameters (7 to 8 mm), bordered by the optic disc nasally and the temporal vascular arcades superiorly and inferiorly (**Fig. 2.1**). Temporally, the macula extends for approximately 2.5 disc diameters (15 degrees) from its center (**Fig. 2.2**). Histologically, the macula is the thickest part of the retina, with more than one layer of ganglion cells. Parallel striations of the nerve fiber layer are visible in an arcuate pattern above and below the macula. The nerve fibers of the central macular region run horizontally toward the optic disc.

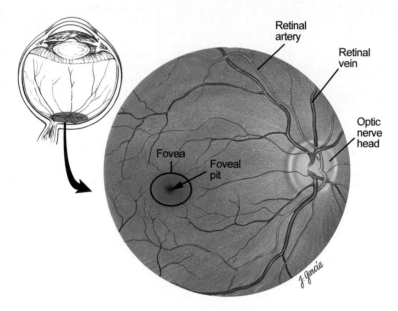

Fig. 2.1 Macula and optic disc. The macula extends for 5 disc diameters (DD) temporal to the optic disc. It is bounded by the superior and inferior vascular arcades. The fovea is the central part of the macula, located 2.5 DD temporal and 0.5 DD inferior to the optic disc. (Drawing by Juan R. Garcia. Used with permission from Johns Hopkins University.)

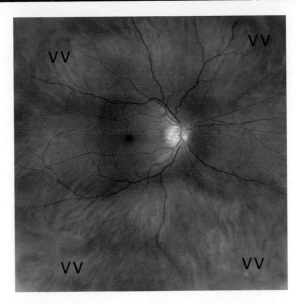

Fig. 2.2   Color fundus photograph showing a wide-angle view of the posterior pole and the equator as marked by the opening of the vortex veins (VV). The fovea is seen as the darker, avascular, central part of the macula.

The fovea is the central part of the macula and corresponds to the site of highest visual acuity. It is approximately 1.5 mm (5 degrees) in size. The central part of the macula, including the fovea, appears darker in color than the surrounding area due to the presence of xanthine and lutein, numerous choriocapillaries, and an increased pigment content of the underlying retinal pigment epithelium (RPE). The center of the fovea, the foveola, measures approximately 350 μm. The foveola is slightly depressed due to the absence of the ganglion cell and inner nuclear layers.

◆ The Optic Disc

Optic disc measures approximately 1700 μm (6 degrees) and is located 4 mm (2.5 disc diameters) nasal to the fovea. It contains the central retinal artery and vein as they branch, a central excavation (cup), and a peripheral neural rim. Normally, the cup/disc ratio is less than 0.6. The cup is located temporal to the entry of the disc vessels.

The normal optic disc is yellow/pink in color. It has clear and well-defined margins, and is at the same plane as the retina (**Fig. 2.3**). Pathologic findings include pallor (atrophy), swelling, and enlarged cupping.

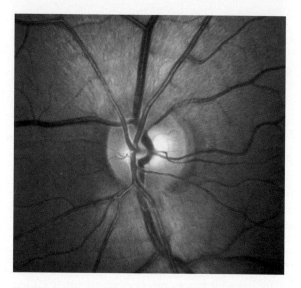

Fig. 2.3 High magnification photograph of a normal left optic disc illustrating physiologic cupping, surface capillaries, and distinct margins. The cup is located temporal to the entry of the disc vessels.

◆ The Equator and Peripheral Fundus

Clinically, the equator of the fundus is defined as the area that includes the internal opening of the vortex veins. The peripheral retina extends from the equator anteriorly to the ora serrata (**Fig. 2.4**).

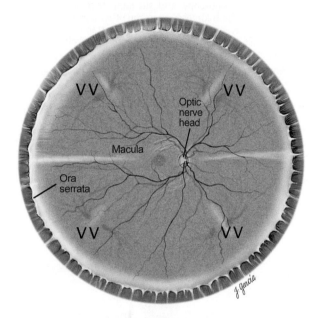

Fig. 2.4 Diagram showing the landmarks of fundus. Peripheral fundus is arbitrarily defined as the area extending anteriorly from the opening of the vortex veins (V V) to the ora serrata. (Drawing by Juan R. Garcia. Used with permission from Johns Hopkins University.)

◆ Common Age-Related Changes in the Fundus

- ◆ Diminished foveal light reflex
- ◆ Drusen, which may develop in the macula or the periphery
- ◆ Minor areas of RPE atrophy
- ◆ Minor pigment clumping in macular region
- ◆ Mild attenuation of retinal vessels
- ◆ Peripheral reticular pigmentary changes
- ◆ Peripheral paving-stone degeneration
- ◆ Vitreous liquefaction and floaters
- ◆ Posterior vitreous detachment

3 Ophthalmoscopy Made Simple

There are several ways to visualize the retina, including direct ophthalmoscopy, binocular indirect ophthalmoscopy, and slit-lamp biomicroscopy. Most general physicians prefer direct ophthalmoscopy to the other methods, because the technique is simple to master, and the device is very portable. Ophthalmologists and optometrists often use slit-lamp biomicroscopy and indirect ophthalmoscopy to obtain a more extensive view of the fundus.

◆ Direct Ophthalmoscope

Direct ophthalmoscopes are simple devices that include a small light source, a viewing aperture, through which the examiner looks at the retina, and a lens dial used for compensating for the examiner's and the patient's refractive errors (**Fig. 3.1**). A recent design, the PanOptic ophthalmoscope (Welch Allyn, Skaneateles Falls, NY), provides a wider field of view.

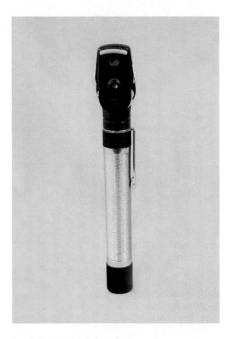

Fig. 3.1   Direct ophthalmoscope.

The advantages of direct ophthalmoscopy:

◆ Simple to use
◆ Upright image
◆ High magnification
◆ Very portable
◆ Relatively low cost

The disadvantages of direct ophthalmoscopy:

◆ No stereoscopic view
◆ Relatively narrow field of view (5 degrees for a standard direct ophthalmoscope and 25 degrees for the PanOptic ophthalmoscope)
◆ Peripheral fundus examination is challenging
◆ Visualization is degraded by the presence of media opacities

How to Use a Direct Ophthalmoscope (Fig. 3.2)

Good alignment is the key to easy, efficient, and rewarding ophthalmoscopy. The goal is to align the examiner's eye with the viewing aperture of the ophthalmoscope, the patient's pupil, and the area of interest on the retina. Both the patient and the examiner should be in a comfortable position (sitting or lying for the patient, sitting or standing for the examiner). Dilating the pupil makes the examination easier.

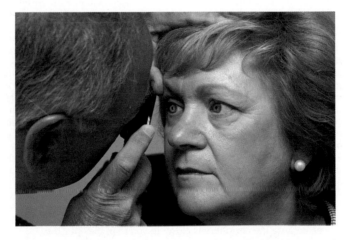

Fig. 3.2 Direct ophthalmoscopy. The examiner uses his right eye and right hand to examine the right eye of the patient. Ideally, the pupils should be dilated.

◆ Instruct the patient to keep the head straight and to look at a distant target straight in front.

◆ Position your head at the same level as the patient's head.

◆ Make yourself and the patient comfortable.

◆ Ask the patient to remove his or her glasses. Contact lenses do not need to be removed. You can keep or remove your glasses.

◆ Use your right eye and right hand to examine the patient's right eye, and your left eye and left hand to examine the patient's left eye.

◆ Dim the room lighting to improve visualization.

◆ Switch the ophthalmoscope on. Use the circular white light, and turn it to maximum to get full illumination.

◆ Examination technique:

  ◦ Using the ophthalmoscope light as a pen light, briefly examine the external features of the eye, including lashes, lid margins, conjunctiva, sclera, iris, and pupil shape, size, and reactivity.

  ◦ Shine the ophthalmoscope light into the patient's pupil at arm's length and observe the red reflex. Note abnormalities of the red reflex such as opacity of the media.

  ◦ Dialing up a +10-diopter (D) lens in the lens wheel, while examining the eye from 10 cm, allows excellent magnification of the anterior segment of the eye.

  ◦ Reduce the power of the lens in the wheel to zero, and move closer to the patient. Identify the optic disc by pointing the ophthalmoscope approximately 15 degrees nasally or by following a blood vessel toward the apex of any branching. If the retina is out of focus, turn the lens dial either way, without moving your head. If the disc becomes clearer, keep turning until the best focus is achieved; if it becomes more blurred, turn the dial the other way.

  ◦ Once you visualize the optic nerve, note its shape, size, color, margins, and the cup, if there is one. Also note the presence of any venous pulsation or surrounding pigment, such as a choroidal or scleral crescent.

  ◦ Next, examine the macula. The macula is the area between the superior and inferior temporal vascular arcades, and its center is the fovea. You can examine the macula by pointing your ophthalmoscope approximately 15 degrees temporal to the optic disc. As an alternative, ask the patient to look into the center of the light. Note the presence or absence of the foveal reflex and the presence of any hemorrhage, exudate, abnormal blood vessel, scar, deposits, or other abnormalities.

  ◦ Examine the retinal blood vessels by re-identifying the optic disc and following each of the four main branches away from the disc. The veins are dark red and relatively large. The arteries are narrower and bright red.

  ◦ Ask the patient to look in the eight cardinal directions to allow you to view the peripheral fundus. In a patient with a well-dilated pupil, it is possible to visualize as far as the equator. You will need to adjust the lens in the focusing wheel, because the periphery is closer to you than the optic disc.

◆ PanOptic Ophthalmoscope

The PanOptic ophthalmoscope (**Fig. 3.3**) is a type of direct ophthalmoscope that is designed to provide a wider view of the fundus. It has a 25-degree field of view, and has slightly more magnification than the standard direct ophthalmoscope. The PanOptic ophthalmoscope can also be used through the undilated pupil.

The advantages of PanOptic ophthalmoscopy are similar to those of the direct ophthalmoscope. An additional advantage over the direct ophthalmoscope is the wider view.

The disadvantages of PanOptic ophthalmoscopy:

◆ Reduced portability
◆ Cost
◆ Monocular viewing limits depth perception

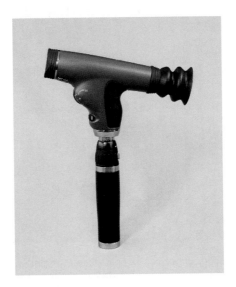

Fig. 3.3   PanOptic ophthalmoscope.

How to Use a PanOptic Ophthalmoscope (Fig. 3.4)

◆ Focus the ophthalmoscope. Look through the scope at an object that is at least 10 to 15 feet away. Focus the scope on the object by using the focusing wheel.
◆ Set aperture dial to "small" or home position.
◆ Turn the scope on, and adjust the light intensity to "maximum."
◆ Instruct the patient to look straight ahead.
◆ Move the ophthalmoscope close to the patient until the eyecup touches the patient's brow. The eyecup should be compressed about half its length to optimize the view.
◆ Visualize the optic disc.
◆ Examine the fundus as described in the section How to Use a Direct Ophthalmoscope (earlier in chapter). The PanOptic ophthalmoscope provides a wider, more panoramic view of the fundus than the standard direct ophthalmoscope.

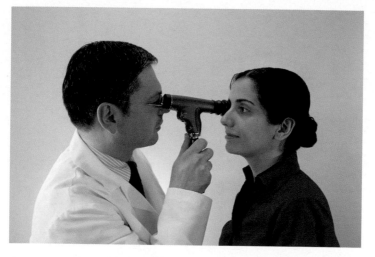

Fig. 3.4 PanOptic ophthalmoscope. The ophthalmoscope is moved close to the patient until the eyecup is compressed about half its length.

◆ Binocular Indirect Ophthalmoscopy

Head-mounted binocular indirect ophthalmoscopy (BIO) is a technique used to evaluate the entire fundus. It provides stereoscopic wide-angle views of the retina and the overlying vitreous. BIO utilizes a head-mounted illumination source, a binocular eyepiece, and a hand-held condensing lens (usually a +20 diopter or +30 diopter lens) (**Fig. 3.5**).

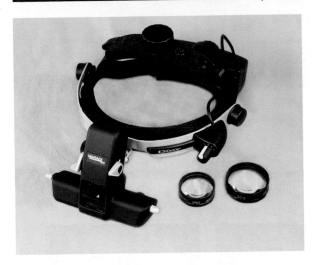

Fig. 3.5   Indirect ophthalmoscope and condensing lenses.

The light beam directed into the patient's eye produces reflected images from the retina and choroid. These images are focused to a viewable, aerial image by the hand-held condensing lens. The resultant image is real, magnified, reversed, and inverted. It is located between the condensing lens and the examiner. The observer views this image through the binocular eyepiece of the head-mounted indirect ophthalmoscope (**Fig. 3.6**). This technique is used by ophthalmologists and optometrists to examine the peripheral retina.

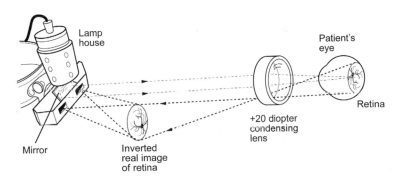

Fig. 3.6   Binocular indirect ophthalmoscope. The condensing lens produces an inverted real image of the patient's retina in a location between the condensing lens and the examiner. The examiner views this image through a binocular eyepiece. (Diagram is not to scale.)

The advantages of indirect ophthalmoscopy:

◆ Stereoscopic view
◆ Wide angle (**Fig. 3.7**)
◆ Superior for peripheral fundus examination
◆ Can be used with scleral depression technique, visualizing the far periphery
◆ Allows visualization of the fundus despite high refractive errors and hazy ocular media

The disadvantages of indirect ophthalmoscopy:

◆ Low magnification
◆ Pupil dilation is essential
◆ The image is inverted and reversed
◆ Takes experience and expertise
◆ Equipment is less portable and more costly than the direct ophthalmoscope

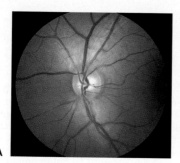 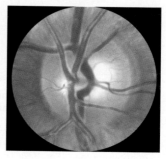

A **B**

Fig. 3.7 The field of vision as seen through an indirect ophthalmoscope (**A**) compared with that seen through a direct ophthalmoscope (**B**).

How to Use a Head-Mounted Binocular Indirect Ophthalmoscope (Fig. 3.8)

◆ Dilate the pupil.
◆ Adjust and secure the head-mount and eyepiece.
◆ Hold a +20 D or a +30 D condensing lens with the thumb, index, and middle fingers approximately 5 cm from the patient's eye, with the more convex surface toward you and the white-ringed edge facing the patient.
◆ From a working distance of 18 to 20 inches, direct the light beam into the pupil, producing a complete red pupillary reflex.
◆ Pull backward on the lens toward you, maintaining the central position of the pupil image, until the entire lens fills with the fundus image.
◆ Make fine adjustments in the lens tilt and distance to the eye to produce a distortion-free full lens view.
◆ For viewing the peripheral fundus, instruct the patient to look in the desired direction, and aim the light beam in that direction, while holding the condensing lens perpendicular to the light beam.

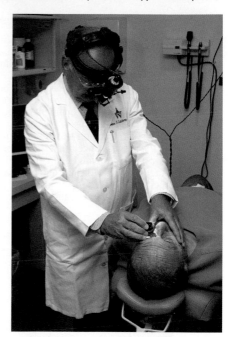

Fig. 3.8 Indirect ophthalmoscopy. The examiner's eyes, eyepiece of ophthalmoscope, the condensing lens, the patient's pupil, and the area of interest on the retina are aligned; the condensing lens is held approximately 5 cm from the patient's eye and moved slightly until the image is focused.

◆ Slit-Lamp Ophthalmoscopy

Slit-lamp ophthalmoscopy utilizes the slit lamp, a horizontally oriented clinical microscope, as the eyepiece, and a condensing lens that may be a contact or noncontact lens.

The advantages of slit-lamp ophthalmoscopy:

◆ Stereoscopic view
◆ High magnification and bright illumination
◆ Variable viewing field, depending on the type of condensing lens
◆ Superior for detailed examination of the optic disc and macula

The disadvantages of slit-lamp ophthalmoscopy:

◆ High cost of equipment
◆ Image may be inverted and reversed depending on the type of condensing lens
◆ Requires experience and expertise
◆ Typically, not portable

How to Perform a Slit-Lamp Ophthalmoscopy (Fig. 3.9)

◆ Dilate the pupil.
◆ Make the patient and yourself comfortable at the slit lamp.
◆ Adjust the optics of the slit lamp, taking into account your interpupillary distance and refraction.
◆ Set the illumination arm of the slit lamp to be coaxial with the viewing system.
◆ Narrow the beam to 1 to 2 mm width with a height corresponding to the diameter of the pupil. Center the beam on the pupil, and focus on the cornea.
◆ Position the condensing lens.
◆ Using the joystick, focus on the fundus image by slowly moving the slit-lamp away from the cornea. Once the retina comes into focus, you can alter the magnification or the light beam height and width to obtain a better image.
◆ Examine the optic disc, macula, and blood vessels.
◆ To view the peripheral retina, instruct the patient to look in the desired direction. It will be necessary to realign the lens and refocus the slit lamp.

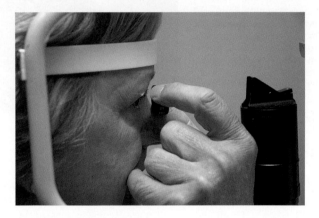

Fig. 3.9   Slit-lamp ophthalmoscopy.

4 Dilation of Pupil

Why dilate the pupil? Dilating the pupil permits a more detailed and efficient fundus examination. It not only provides a better view of the optic disc and macula, but also makes it possible to examine the peripheral retina.

◆ How to Dilate the Pupil

One drop of tropicamide 1% often achieves enough pupillary dilation to allow routine screening examination in most cases. Maximal pupil dilation is often required for detailed examination of the peripheral retina. This is usually achieved by a combination of one drop of phenylephrine 2.5% and either tropicamide 1% or cyclopentolate 1%. The drops can be repeated 2–3 times, every 5–10 minutes, if the pupil does not dilate well. The pupils of blue-eyed patients dilate more quickly than the pupils of brown-eyed patients.

- ◆ Tropicamide 1%—onset of action 15 minutes; duration 2 to 4 hours
- ◆ Cyclopentolate 1%—onset 20 minutes; duration 4 to 6 hours
- ◆ Phenylephrine 2.5%—onset 20 minutes; duration 4 to 6 hours. Phenylephrine is used in conjunction with tropicamide or cyclopentolate for maximum dilation of the pupil.

◆ Concerns About Pupillary Dilation

- ◆ Blurred vision—After pupillary dilation, the vision becomes blurred, mainly for close-up work, such as reading. In some patients the distance vision may also become affected. In these patients the vision usually recovers enough for driving within 2 hours.
- ◆ Light sensitivity—Pupillary dilation often causes mild and transient light sensitivity that is relieved by wearing sunglasses.
- ◆ Angle closure glaucoma—Acute angle closure glaucoma rarely occurs after pupillary dilation. Advise the patient of symptoms of pain and redness occurring within 24 hours of dilation of the pupil. The pain may be in the eye, or in the forehead, or elsewhere in the head.
- ◆ Neurologic/neurosurgical patient—Pupillary dilation may interfere with neurological evaluation, for example, for head injury. Dilated ophthalmoscopy in these patients should be performed only after discussion with the neurosurgery team.

5 Pearls

◆ During direct ophthalmoscopy:
- ○ It is advisable for the examiner to keep both eyes open and mentally suppress the image from the other eye.
- ○ The closer you are to the patient, the better is your visualization of the fundus, as both the field of vision and illumination improve.
- ○ The power of lens necessary to focus on the fundus depends on both the patient's and the examiner's refractive error and accommodation.
- ○ The optic disc is the main landmark when visualizing the fundus. It is situated 15 degrees nasal to the visual axis. Knowing this fact helps in rapid identification of the optic disc. Start your fundus visualization by instructing the patient to look straight ahead, and then direct the ophthalmoscope 15 degrees nasally. The optic disc will be directly in front of you.
- ○ To visualize the macula, instruct the patient to look directly at the center of the light, or at the fixation target that is built into most direct ophthalmoscopes.
- ○ Some direct ophthalmoscopes have a grid incorporated into their illumination dial. The size of a small posteriorly located lesion can be compared with the size of the optic disc by utilizing this grid (**Fig. 5.1**).

Aperture	Description	Use
○	Full size	Observing through large pupil
○	Small size	Observing through small pupil
●	Red-free (green) filter	Assists in detecting abnormalities in the nerve fiber layer and in observing microaneurysms and other red vascular lesions
❙	Slit beam	Judging retinal contour
⊞	Reticule	Measuring vessel caliber or diameter of a small retinal lesion (marked in increments of tenths of mm)
⊗	Fixation target	Aligning observer's own macula with fixating portion of patient's macula (normally the foveal pit)

Fig. 5.1 Various apertures are available in most direct ophthalmoscopes. Modified from: *Practical Ophthalmology. A Manual for Beginning Residents.* Editor: Fred M. Wilson (4th edition). American Academy of Ophthalmology. 1996.

° Follow a routine sequence: external eye, red reflex, anterior segment, disc, vessels, macula, and periphery.

◆ Using the red-free (green) light improves contrast and allows better visualization of the optic nerve fiber layer and hemorrhages (**Fig. 5.2**).

◆ The size of any retinal lesion can be estimated by comparing it with the optic disc (approximately 1700 μm), or a retinal vein as it crosses the disc margin (approximately 125 μm).

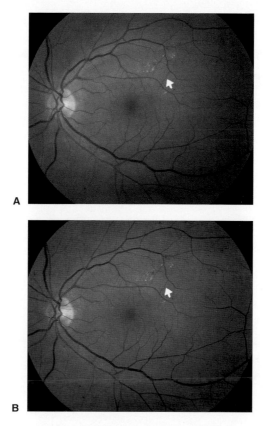

Fig. 5.2 Red lesions such as blood vessels and hemorrhages (*arrows*) (**A**) are better visualized by using the red-free (green) filter (**B**).

II
Clinical Signs in the Retina and Differential Diagnosis

◆ Types of Retinal Hemorrhages

◆ Superficial flame-shaped hemorrhages (**Fig. 6.1**)
  ∘ Located at the level of superficial nerve fiber layer; represents hemorrhage from the inner capillary network of the retina

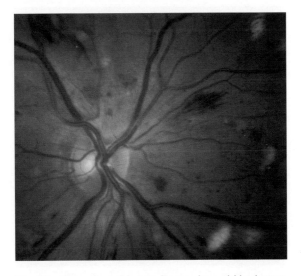

Fig. 6.1 Flame-shaped hemorrhages, dot and blot hemorrhages, and cotton-wool spots (CWSs) in a patient with severe nonproliferative diabetic retinopathy.

◆ White-centered hemorrhages (**Fig. 6.2**)
  ◦ A white-centered hemorrhage is a superficial flame-shaped hemorrhage with an area of central whitening, often representing focal necrosis or cellular infiltration. Causes of white-centered hemorrhage include bacterial endocarditis and septicemia (Roth spots), lymphoproliferative disorders, diabetes mellitus, hypertension, anemia, collagen vascular disorders, and scurvy.
◆ Dot hemorrhages (**Fig. 6.3**)
  ◦ Small, round, and superficial hemorrhage; represent hemorrhages from the superficial capillary network of the retina; clinically resembles microaneurysms
◆ Blot hemorrhages (**Fig. 6.4**)
  ◦ Medium size, dark, and intraretinal; represent hemorrhaging from the deep capillary network of the retina

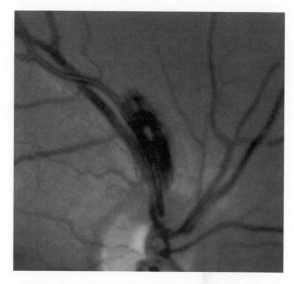

Fig. 6.2   White-centered hemorrhage (Roth spot).

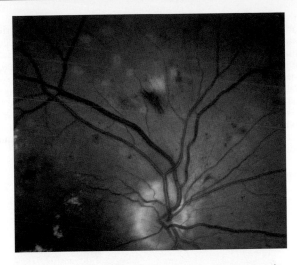

Fig. 6.3 Multiple dot hemorrhages are present superonasal to the optic disc. Old laser photocoagulation scars (superior to the disc) and hard exudates (temporal to the disc) are present.

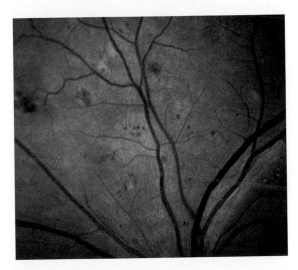

Fig. 6.4 Dot hemorrhages are small, well-circumscribed, and bright red lesions. Blot hemorrhages are larger dark red lesions with slightly fuzzy margins, resembling an "ink-blot."

◆ Retrohyaloid hemorrhage (**Fig. 6.5**)
  ◦ Variable in size; may have "fluid level" ("boat-shaped" hemorrhage); located anterior (internal) to the retina, within the retrohyaloid space
◆ Subretinal hemorrhage (**Fig. 6.6**)
  ◦ Located deep (external) to the retina; variable in size. The retinal vessels can be seen crossing over (internal to) the hemorrhage. Subretinal hemorrhages are variable in size and most commonly are caused by choroidal neovascularization, for example, exudative ("wet") macular degeneration.
◆ Vitreous hemorrhage
  ◦ Intravitreal hemorrhage, most commonly caused by a retinal lesion; may be localized or diffuse, and also occurs in association with elevated intracranial pressure; e.g., Terson's syndrome.

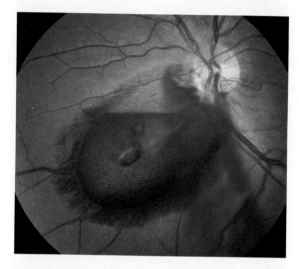

Fig. 6.5 Retrohyaloid and intravitreal hemorrhage in a patient with Valsalva retinopathy. Retrohyaloid hemorrhage is located within the space between the inner surface of the retina and the posterior hyaloid face. The upper border is usually straight with a "fluid level"; it obscures the retinal blood vessels, which run posterior (deep) to it.

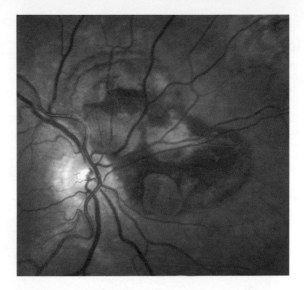

Fig. 6.6 Subretinal hemorrhage in a patient with exudative "wet" age-related macular degeneration. The hemorrhage is located deep to the retina. The retinal vessels are seen passing over the area of subretinal hemorrhage.

Conditions Associated with Retinal Hemorrhages

- Diabetic retinopathy
- Systemic hypertension
- Retinal vein occlusion
- Retinal artery occlusion—typically causes less hemorrhage than vein occlusion
- Carotid artery disease
- Sickle cell retinopathy
- Radiation retinopathy
- HIV retinopathy
- Retinitis (e.g., cytomegalovirus retinitis in patients with AIDS)
- Retinal macroaneurysm
- Retinal vasculitis
- Shaken baby syndrome
- Anemia
- Lymphoproliferative disorders
- Coagulopathy
- Hyperviscosity
- Papilledema
- Endocarditis
- Septicemia
- Terson's syndrome
- Valsalva retinopathy
- Purtscher retinopathy
- Trauma
  - Ocular injury
  - Head injury
  - Compression injuries of chest and abdomen
- Age-related macular degeneration
- Posterior vitreous detachment

7 Hard Exudates

Hard exudates (HEs) are well-circumscribed shiny, yellow deposits that are usually located deep to the superficial retinal vessels, within the retina in the outer plexiform layer (**Fig. 7.1**). They arise at the margins of areas of retinal edema and indicate abnormal capillary permeability. HEs contain lipoproteins and lipid-laden macrophages. They may clear spontaneously or after laser photocoagulation of leaking blood vessels, often within 6 months.

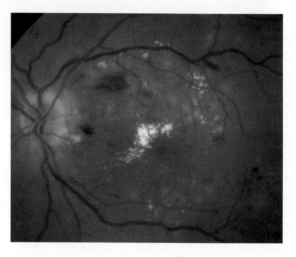

Fig. 7.1 Hard exudates are yellow shiny deposits that are usually located within the retina. Hard exudates are a sign of chronic retinal edema and vascular leakage.

Patterns of Hard Exudates

◆ Isolated, scattered.
◆ Circinate pattern (**Fig. 7.2**)—complete or partial circle of HEs surround an area of retinal edema. The central area often contains leaking microaneurysms and is the site of maximal leakage.
◆ Macular star (**Fig. 7.3**)—Radiating star-shaped pattern of HEs is seen in diabetic retinopathy, severe systemic hypertension, papilledema, and neuroretinitis associated with cat-scratch and other diseases.
◆ Subretinal hard exudates (**Fig. 7.4**)—Subretinal HEs are most commonly associated with choroidal neovascularization in exudative (wet) macular degeneration. They may also be seen in severe, chronic diabetic maculopathy.

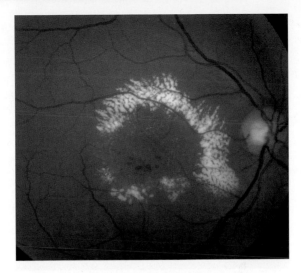

Fig. 7.2 Circinate pattern of hard exudates in a patient with retinal telangiectasis. The exudates surround an area of retinal edema, leaking microaneurysms, and telangiectatic vessels.

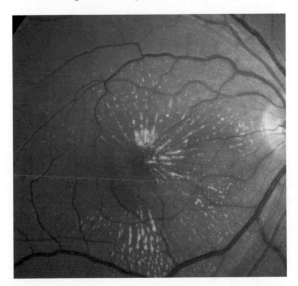

Fig. 7.3 Macular star—hard exudates in a radial "star-shaped" pattern in a patient with severe systemic hypertension.

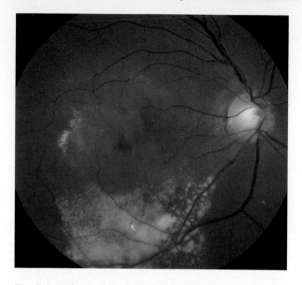

Fig. 7.4 Subretinal hard exudates in exudative "wet" age-related macular degeneration.

Conditions Associated with Hard Exudates (HE)

HEs can occur in any condition that causes retinal and optic nerve microvascular leakage:
♦ Diabetic retinopathy
♦ Systemic hypertension
♦ Retinal vein occlusion
♦ Papilledema
♦ Radiation retinopathy
♦ Retinal vasculitis
♦ Neuroretinitis (e.g., cat-scratch disease, Lyme disease)
♦ Retinal vascular lesions
  ◦ Macroaneurysm
  ◦ Capillary hemangioma (von Hippel–Lindau disease)
  ◦ Coats disease
  ◦ Idiopathic parafoveal telangiectasia
♦ Choroidal tumors—malignant melanoma, metastasis
♦ Hyperviscosity syndromes
♦ Serous retinal detachment
♦ Age-related macular degeneration

Lesions that May Resemble Hard Exudates

◆ Drusen—yellow or cream-colored, subretinal deposits that often have blurred margins. They are usually seen alone or in association with age-related macular degeneration. Unlike HEs, drusen are not usually shiny or refractile. Calcified drusen, however, may appear refractile (**Fig. 7.5**).

◆ Retinal and subretinal deposits; e.g., canthaxanthine, tamoxifen.

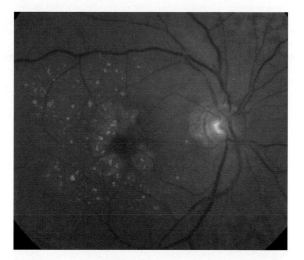

Fig. 7.5   Calcified drusen—multiple refractile deposits resembling hard exudates in a patient with dry age-related macular degeneration. An area of geographic atrophy is present. There are no signs of retinal vasculopathy. Typical nonrefractile (noncalcified) drusen are present temporal to the area of geographic atrophy.

Microaneurysms are fusiform or saccular outpouchings of the retinal capillaries. They appear as red dots (similar to dot hemorrhages), measuring 15 to 50 μm (**Fig. 8.1**). They represent microvasculopathy of the retina and develop secondary to capillary wall weakness that results from loss of supporting pericytes. Microaneurysms have increased permeability and may bleed or leak, resulting in retinal hemorrhage or edema. The natural history of a microaneurysm includes initial increase in size and leakage, followed by a decrease in size and reduced leakage. Thrombosis and occlusion of microaneurysm lead to their disappearance within 3 to 6 months.

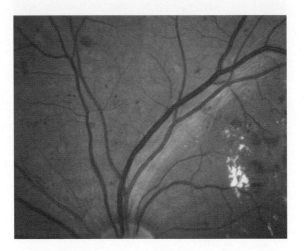

Fig. 8.1 Microaneurysms are small, well-circumscribed, red, intraretinal lesions that resemble dot hemorrhages. They represent retinal microvasculopathy. Distinction between microaneurysms and dot hemorrhages can be difficult, but is usually of no clinical significance.

Conditions Associated with Microaneurysms

◆ Diabetic retinopathy
◆ Hypertension
◆ Retinal vein occlusion
◆ Carotid artery disease
◆ Radiation retinopathy
◆ Vasculitis
◆ Anemia
◆ Thrombocytopenia
◆ Lymphoproliferative disorders
◆ Hyperviscosity
◆ Purtscher retinopathy

9 Cotton-Wool Spots

Cotton-wool spots (CWSs) are yellow-white superficial retinal lesions with characteristic indistinct feathery borders measuring between 0.25 and 1 disc diameter in size (**Fig. 9.1**). CWSs represent areas of extra- and intraaxonal swelling within the retinal nerve fiber layer due to focal ischemia. They are often associated with areas of capillary nonperfusion. CWSs usually resolve spontaneously within 3 months. If the underlying condition persists, new lesions develop in different locations.

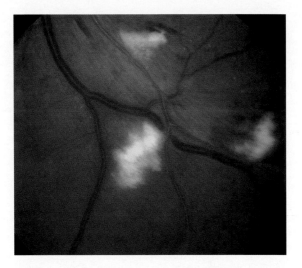

Fig. 9.1 Cotton-wool spots are yellow-white lesions with feathery borders, located within the superficial nerve fiber layer. They represent focal areas of ischemia.

Conditions Associated with Cotton-Wool Spots

- Diabetic retinopathy
- Hypertensive retinopathy (**Fig. 9.2**)
- HIV
- Systemic lupus erythematosus (SLE) and other collagen vascular disorders
- Retinal vein occlusion
- Retinal artery occlusion
- Microemboli/septic emboli
- Carotid artery stenosis
- Radiation retinopathy
- Hyperviscosity syndromes
- Anemia
- Leukemia and other lymphoproliferative disorders
- Retinal vasculitis
- Purtscher/Purtscher-like retinopathy
- Ocular trauma
- Interferon therapy

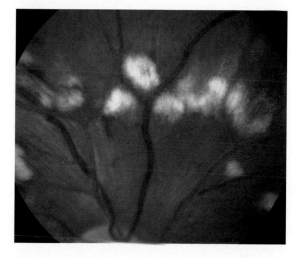

Fig. 9.2   Multiple cotton-wool spots in a patient with severe hypertension.

Lesions Resembling Cotton-Wool Spots

◆ Myelinated nerve fiber layer (**Fig. 9.3**)
◆ Early cytomegalovirus (CMV) retinitis
◆ Retinal infiltrates (e.g., candida)

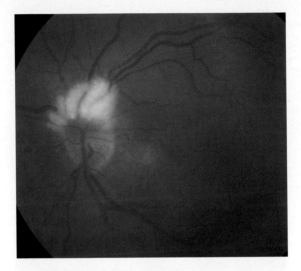

Fig. 9.3 Myelinated nerve fibers (MNFs)—yellow-white lesion superior to the optic disc. MNFs have feathery margins, and may resemble cotton-wool spots. Unlike CWSs, MNFs do not resolve.

Retinal edema manifests as increased retinal thickness (**Fig. 10.1**) that is best visualized by slit-lamp ophthalmoscopy. Hard exudates are often present adjacent to or within the area of edema. Retinal edema is due to breakdown in the blood–retinal barrier, resulting in abnormal leakage from the retinal vasculature. The physiologic processes involved in removing fluid from the retina are overcome by the excessive leakage from abnormal blood vessels and microaneurysms, resulting in retinal edema. Another mechanism for development of retinal edema is ischemic swelling of the retinal tissue.

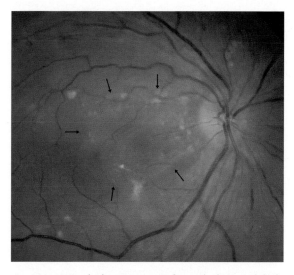

Fig. 10.1 Retinal edema. An area of retinal edema and thickening is present between the optic disc and the fovea (*arrows*) in a patient with severe systemic hypertension. Fine hard exudates can be seen near the inferotemporal and temporal border of edematous and nonedematous retina. Multiple small cotton-wool spots are present.

Conditions Associated with Focal or Diffuse Retinal Edema

◆ Diabetic retinopathy
◆ Hypertension
◆ Retinal vein occlusion
◆ Retinal artery occlusion—ischemic cloudy swelling, rather than true edema
◆ Retinal macroaneurysms
◆ Retinal vascular malformations
◆ Other forms of retinal vasculopathy
◆ Hyperviscosity
◆ Papilledema
◆ Neuroretinitis—Lyme disease, cat-scratch disease, syphilis
◆ Ocular trauma—commotio retinae
◆ Age-related macular degeneration

Conditions Associated with Cystoid Macular Edema

◆ Intraocular surgery
◆ Diabetic retinopathy
◆ Retinal vein occlusion
◆ Intraocular inflammation
◆ Retinitis pigmentosa
◆ Vitreomacular traction
◆ Age-related macular degeneration
◆ Drugs—niacin, epinephrine, dipivefrin, latanoprost
◆ Autosomal dominant cystoid macular edema

11 Retinal Neovascularization

Retinal neovascular complexes are abnormal meshworks of fine blood vessels that grow in response to severe retinal ischemia or chronic inflammation. They may occur on or adjacent to the optic disc (neovascularization at the disc [NVD]) (**Figs. 11.1, 11.2, and 11.3**) or elsewhere in the retina (neovascularization elsewhere [NVE]) (**Figs. 11.4 and 11.5**). Neovascular complexes may be flat on the retina or protrude into the vitreous. NVD and any elevated neovascularization (NV) tend to have a high risk for hemorrhage.

Conditions Associated with Retinal Neovascularization

◆ Proliferative diabetic retinopathy
◆ Proliferative sickle cell retinopathy
◆ Retinal vein occlusion
◆ Retinal artery occlusion
◆ Microemboli (e.g., talc retinopathy secondary to intravenous drug abuse)
◆ Retinopathy of prematurity
◆ Retinal vasculitis
◆ Carotid artery stenosis
◆ Aortic arch syndrome
◆ Carotid-cavernous fistula
◆ Hyperviscosity syndromes (e.g., chronic leukemia)
◆ Ocular/periocular irradiation
◆ Intraocular tumors
◆ Intraocular inflammation—sarcoidosis, pars planitis, bird-shot chorioretinopathy, chronic uveitis
◆ Chronic retinal detachment
◆ Familial exudative vitreoretinopathy (FEVR)
◆ Incontinentia pigmenti
◆ Norrie's disease

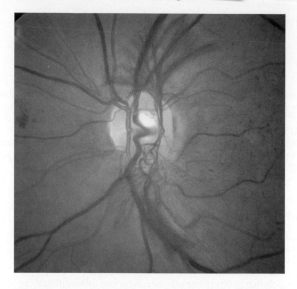

Fig. 11.1 Neovascularization at the disc (NVD). Fine neovascular fronds are seen originating from the optic disc in this patient with proliferative diabetic retinopathy.

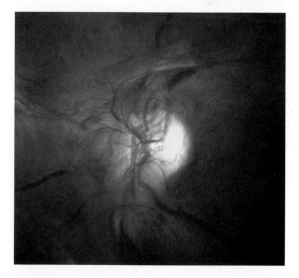

Fig. 11.2 Neovascularization at the disc (NVD). Severe NVD extending superiorly, nasally, and inferiorly, with early underlying tractional retinal detachment.

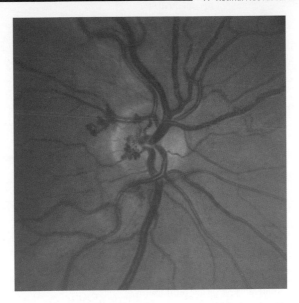

Fig. 11.3 Regressed neovascularization at the disc (NVD). The vascular meshwork consists of larger-caliber vessels, and has lost the fine marginal fronds that are characteristic of active new vessel complexes.

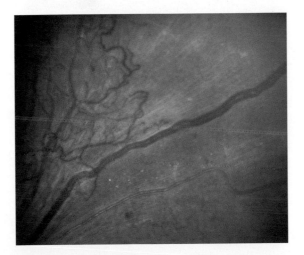

Fig. 11.4 Neovascularization elsewhere (NVE). Large NVE in a patient with proliferative diabetic retinopathy (top left). Note the featureless and avascular area of retina distal to the NVE (top right). Venous beading is present.

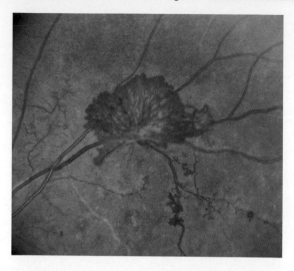

Fig. 11.5   "Sea-fan" neovascularization (NVE) in a patient with proliferative sickle cell retinopathy.

12 Iris Neovascularization

Iris neovascularization (rubeosis iridis) is characterized by the presence of fine networks of abnormal blood vessels over the iris surface and at the margin of the pupil (**Fig. 12.1**). It arises as a response to abnormally elevated concentrations of angiogenic factors, often due to ischemia of the retina or the anterior segment. Iris neovascularization is a serious complication of ocular ischemia and may lead to angle closure and severe intractable glaucoma, resulting in a blind painful eye. Spontaneous bleeding (hyphema) may occur.

Conditions Associated with Iris Neovascularization

◆ Advanced diabetic eye disease
◆ Retinal vein occlusion
◆ Retinal artery occlusion
◆ Carotid artery stenosis
◆ Aortic arch syndrome
◆ Carotid-cavernous fistula
◆ Giant cell arteritis
◆ Ocular/periocular irradiation
◆ Intraocular tumors
◆ Intraocular inflammation
◆ Anterior segment ischemia
  ◦ Anterior segment ischemia can occur in sickle cell disease, giant cell arteritis, severe carotid stenosis, and following extensive strabismus and retinal detachment surgery.

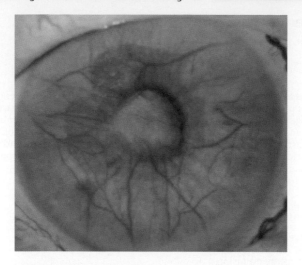

Fig. 12.1 Neovascularization of the iris (NVI) (rubeosis) is seen in a patient with advanced diabetic eye disease.

13 Retinal Emboli

Types of Retinal Emboli

◆ Platelet emboli (**Fig. 13.1**) are soft and grayish white in appearance, and conform to the shape of the blood vessel. They usually originate from an ulcerating atheromatous plaque within the carotid artery and can cause amaurosis fugax. They may be seen moving along the retinal vasculature.

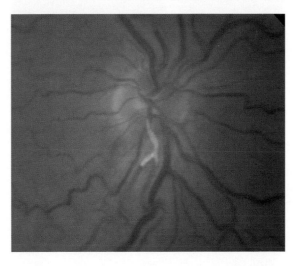

Fig. 13.1 Platelet emboli—soft, grayish white platelet emboli conforming to the shape of the blood vessel. Vascular tortuosity is due to coexisting, chronic systemic hypertension.

◆ Cholesterol emboli—Hollenhorst plaques are yellow crystalline deposits that are commonly found at the bifurcations of the retinal arteries. They may cause transient occlusion of blood flow, resulting in transient loss of vision (amaurosis fugax). They often signify atheromatous disease of the carotid artery.

◆ Calcific emboli (**Figs. 13.2 and 13.3**) have a pearly white appearance, are often larger than the platelet and cholesterol emboli, and tend to lodge in the larger retinal arteries around the optic disc. Calcific emboli usually occlude blood flow and can be visually symptomatic. They often originate from the aortic or mitral valve.

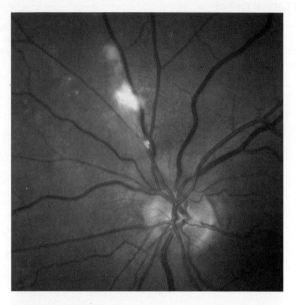

Fig. 13.2 Calcific embolus—yellow-white calcific embolus occluding a superonasal retinal artery. Note attenuation of the arteriole distal to the site of occlusion, and cotton-wool spots (CWSs).

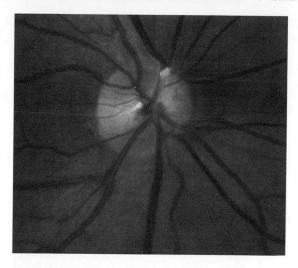

Fig. 13.3 Refractile, yellow-white, calcific embolus in a patient with a history of carotid artery disease.

◆ Septic emboli can cause white-centered retinal hemorrhages (Roth spots), retinal microabscesses, and endogenous endophthalmitis.
◆ Fat emboli can cause Purtscher-like retinopathy.
◆ Amniotic fluid emboli can cause Purtscher-like retinopathy.
◆ Talc emboli are seen in intravenous drug abuse.
◆ Tumor emboli are rare.

Sources of Retinal Emboli

◆ Carotid artery atheromatous plaque
◆ Cardiac valve abnormalities
◆ Cardiac defects
◆ Atrial myxoma
◆ Bacterial endocarditis/septicemia/fungemia
◆ Intravenous drugs

14 Retinal Crystal Deposition

Retinal crystals appear as multiple, fine, refractile, yellow-white deposits (**Figs. 14.1, 14.2 and 14.3**).

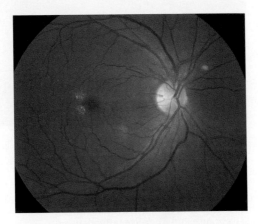

Fig. 14.1 Crystalline deposits—fine, juxtafoveal intraretinal crystalline deposits in a patient with idiopathic juxtafoveal telangiectasis. Note the gray reflex and telangiectasis in the central macular region.

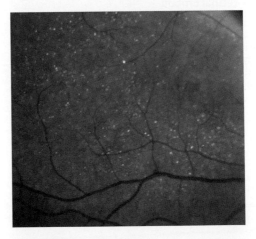

Fig. 14.2 Crystalline deposits—multiple, refractile, retinal deposits in a patient with cystinosis.

Differential Diagnosis

◆ Systemic disorders
  ◦ Cystinosis—infantile variety
  ◦ Primary hyperoxaluria
  ◦ Secondary oxalosis
  ◦ Sjögren-Larson syndrome
  ◦ Microemboli
  ◦ Intravenous drug abuse—talc retinopathy (**Fig. 14.3**)
◆ Drugs
  ◦ Tamoxifen
  ◦ Canthaxanthine
  ◦ Nitrofurantoin
  ◦ Methoxyfluorane
  ◦ Ethylene glycol ingestion
◆ Ocular conditions
  ◦ Juxtafoveal telangiectasis, Type II
  ◦ Gyrate atrophy
  ◦ Bietti crystalline degeneration
  ◦ Calcified drusen

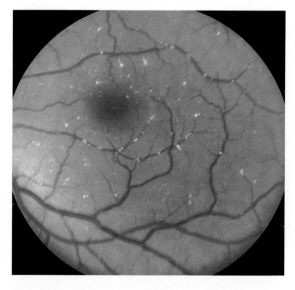

Fig. 14.3 White, refractile, crystalline deposits primarily at retinal vessels, characteristic of talc retinopathy in a patient with a history of intravenous drug abuse.

15 Retinal Vascular Sheathing

Vascular sheathing is the appearance of a yellow-white cuff or sheath surrounding part or all of a retinal artery or vein (**Figs. 15.1 and 15.2**).

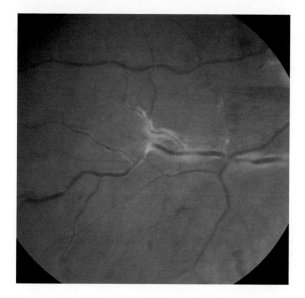

Fig. 15.1 Vascular sheathing—whitish sheathing of retinal vessels in a patient with sarcoidosis. Fine yellow-white intra-retinal infiltrates and hemorrhages are also present.

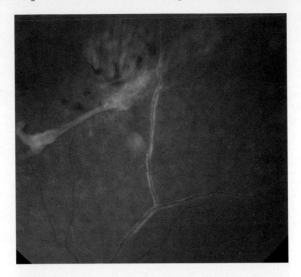

Fig. 15.2 Diffuse venous sheathing in a patient with long-standing branch retinal vein occlusion.

Conditions Associated with Retinal Vascular Sheathing

◆ Sarcoidosis
◆ Multiple sclerosis
◆ Behçet disease
◆ Retinal vasculitis
◆ Systemic hypertension
◆ Old retinal vein occlusion
◆ Chronic leukemia
◆ Amyloidosis
◆ Pars planitis
◆ Infections
  ◦ Tuberculosis
  ◦ Syphilis
  ◦ Toxoplasmosis
  ◦ Lyme disease
  ◦ Cat-scratch disease
  ◦ HIV
  ◦ Cytomegalovirus
  ◦ Herpes zoster and herpes simplex

Retinal vascular telangiectasis is abnormal dilatation and tortuosity of small retinal blood vessels (**Fig. 16.1**). It occurs in conditions that cause retinal vasculopathy.

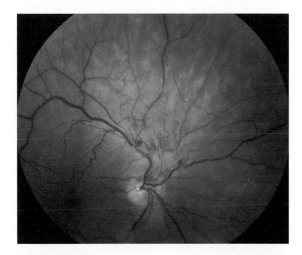

Fig. 16.1 Retinal vascular telangiectasis—multiple dilated and tortuous retinal vessels in the superior quadrant. Sheathing of the retinal vein (superiorly) is suggestive of old branch retinal vein occlusion.

Conditions Associated with Retinal Vascular Telangiectasis

- Diabetes mellitus
- Systemic hypertension
- Retinal vascular occlusion
- Radiation retinopathy
- Sickle cell disease
- Papilledema
- Incontinentia pigmenti
- Leber optic neuropathy
- Tuberous sclerosis
- Alport disease
- Facioscapulohumeral dystrophy
- Epidermal nevus syndrome
- Ocular
  - Coats disease
  - Idiopathic juxtafoveal telangiectasis
  - Chronic retinal detachment
  - Retinitis pigmentosa

Retinal detachment is the separation of the retina from the underlying retinal pigment epithelium (RPE). There are three main types of retinal detachment: (1) serous/exudative, (2) tractional, and (3) rhegmatogenous.

◆ Serous/Exudative Retinal Detachment (Figs. 17.1 and 17.2)

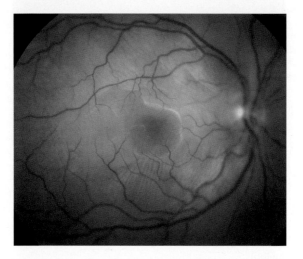

Fig. 17.1 Serous retinal detachment—elevation of the retina, indicated by the increased curvature of the retinal vessels, as well as translucent retina with folds, in a patient with pre-eclampsia.

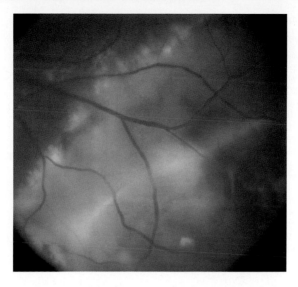

Fig. 17.2 Exudative retinal detachment. The retina is elevated, and retinal and subretinal hard exudates and hemorrhages
are present in this patient with exudative retinal detachment in
Coats disease.

In serous retinal detachment, the surface of the detached retina is smooth, and the
location of the subretinal fluid is position-dependent, characteristically gravitating
to the lowermost part of the fundus (shifting fluid sign). Retinal breaks are absent.

Conditions Associated with Serous/Exudative Retinal Detachment

◆ Severe systemic hypertension
◆ Eclampsia/preeclampsia
◆ Renal failure
◆ Dural arteriovenous shunt
◆ Retinal vascular anomalies
  ◦ Retinal hemangioblastoma (hemangioma)
  ◦ Retinal macroaneurysm
  ◦ Retinal telangiectasia
  ◦ Familial exudative vitreoretinopathy

◆ Inflammatory
  ◦ Posterior scleritis
  ◦ Uveitis
  ◦ Vogt-Koyanagi-Harada disease
  ◦ Connective tissue diseases
  ◦ Neuroretinitis
  ◦ Orbital pseudotumor
◆ Infectious
  ◦ Syphilis
  ◦ Toxoplasma retinochoroiditis
  ◦ Cysticercosis
  ◦ Herpes zoster ophthalmicus
  ◦ Orbital cellulitis
  ◦ Infected scleral buckle
◆ Neoplastic
  ◦ Choroidal malignant melanoma
  ◦ Choroidal metastasis
  ◦ Choroidal hemangioma
  ◦ Combined hamartomas of the retina and retinal pigment epithelium
  ◦ Lymphoma
  ◦ Multiple myeloma
  ◦ Leukemia
◆ Hematologic
  ◦ Hyperviscosity syndromes
  ◦ Disseminated intravascular coagulopathy
◆ Chorioretinal disorders
  ◦ Idiopathic central serous chorioretinopathy
  ◦ Intense panretinal laser photocoagulation
  ◦ Choroidal detachment
  ◦ Choroidal neovascularization
  ◦ Choroidal ischemia (e.g., severe hypertension, embolic disease)
  ◦ Idiopathic uveal effusion syndrome
◆ Optic nerve pit
◆ Papilledema

◆ Tractional Retinal Detachment (Fig. 17.3)

Tractional retinal detachment (TRD) is caused by traction on the retina in the absence of a retinal break. The retina in the area of detachment is immobile and concave forward (anteriorly). The retinal detachment rarely extends to the ora serrata. Fibrovascular proliferation is a frequent associated finding.

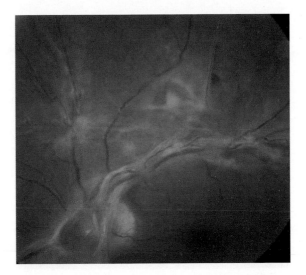

Fig. 17.3   Tractional retinal detachment (TRD)—fibrovascular bands and membranes exerting traction with localized elevation of the retina in a patient with advanced diabetic eye disease.

Conditions Associated with Tractional Retinal Detachment

- ◆ Severe proliferative diabetic retinopathy
- ◆ Retinopathy of prematurity
- ◆ Other vascular proliferative retinopathies—retinal vein occlusion, sickle cell retinopathy, radiation retinopathy, Eales disease, Behçet disease, retinal vasculitis, familial exudative vitreoretinopathy, incontinentia pigmenti
- ◆ Proliferative vitreoretinopathy
- ◆ Recurrent vitreous hemorrhage
- ◆ Trauma
  - ◦ Intraocular foreign body
  - ◦ Vitreous incarceration
- ◆ Intraocular inflammation—chronic vitritis, toxocara chorioretinitis, cysticercosis
- ◆ Persistent fetal vasculature

◆ Rhegmatogenous Retinal Detachment (Fig. 17.4)

Rhegmatogenous retinal detachment (RRD) is caused by the abnormal presence of a retinal break or tear, allowing fluid from the vitreous cavity to gain access to the subretinal space. The surface of the retina is usually convex forward. Rhegmatogenous retinal detachment has a corrugated appearance, and undulates with eye movement. The area of the detached retina usually extends to the ora serrata.

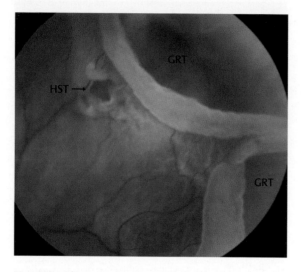

Fig. 17.4 Rhegmatogenous retinal detachment—giant retinal tear (GRT), as well as a horseshoe tear (HST), in a patient with rhegmatogenous retinal detachment. The retina is folded and has hydration lines over the detached area.

Causes of Retinal Breaks

- ◆ Posterior vitreous detachment
- ◆ Severe vitreoretinal traction
- ◆ Trauma
- ◆ Intraocular surgery
- ◆ Retinal necrosis (e.g., cytomegalovirus [CMV] retinitis)
- ◆ Atrophic holes (e.g., associated with degenerative areas in the retina, such as lattice degeneration)

18 Bull's-Eye Maculopathy

Bull's-eye maculopathy is pigmentary degeneration of the macula that occurs in a bull's-eye pattern.

Conditions Associated with Bull's-Eye Maculopathy

◆ Chloroquine/hydroxychloroquine maculopathy (**Fig. 18.1**)
◆ Cone dystrophy
◆ Stargardt disease (**Fig. 18.2**)
◆ Age-related macular degeneration (**Fig. 18.3**)
◆ Tamoxifen retinopathy
◆ Canthaxanthine maculopathy
◆ Phototoxicity
◆ Benign concentric annular macular dystrophy
◆ Adult vitelliform dystrophy; pattern dystrophy
◆ Batten disease
◆ Olivopontocerebellar degeneration
◆ Spielmeyer-Vogt syndrome

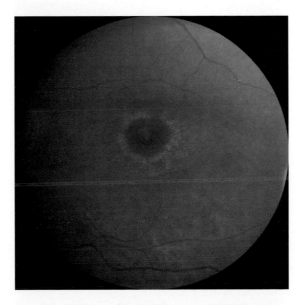

Fig. 18.1 Bull's-eye maculopathy—rings of retinal pigment epithelial atrophy and degeneration centered on the fovea in a "target" or "bull's-eye" pattern in a patient with hydroxychloroquine-associated maculopathy.

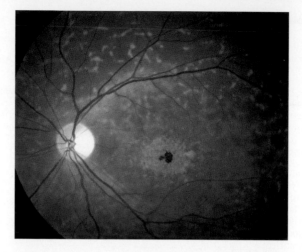

Fig. 18.2 Bull's-eye maculopathy in a patient with Stargardt disease. Subretinal yellow "flecks" are characteristic findings in Stargardt disease.

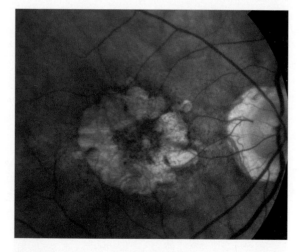

Fig. 18.3 Bull's-eye maculopathy—"target" lesion in a patient with atrophic age-related macular degeneration ("geographic" atrophy).

19 Cherry-Red Spot at the Macula

Cherry-red spot at the macula is the terminology used to describe the dark red appearance of the central foveal area in comparison with the surrounding, abnormal grayish-white macular region (**Fig. 19.1**). This appearance is most commonly due to a relative loss of transparency of the parafoveal retina resulting from ischemic cloudy swelling.

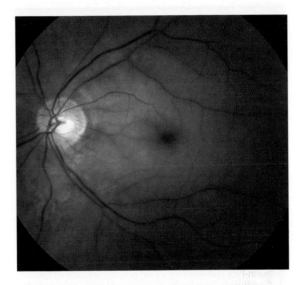

Fig. 19.1 Cherry-red spot at the macula in a patient with recent central retinal artery occlusion. The white-gray appearance of retina is due to diffuse, ischemic cloudy swelling. The dark red appearance of the fovea is due to the transmission of normal choroidal color through the relatively thin retina in the central foveal region.

Differential Diagnosis

◆ Central retinal artery occlusion
◆ Sphingolipidoses
  ◦ Gangliosidoses (Tay-Sachs disease and Sandhoff disease, et al.)
  ◦ Niemann-Pick disease types A to D (**Fig. 19.2**)
  ◦ Metachromatic leukodystrophy
  ◦ Farber disease
◆ Mucopolysaccharidoses
  ◦ Hurler disease
◆ Mucolipidoses; sialidoses

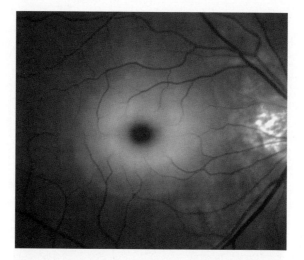

Fig. 19.2 Cherry-red spot at the macula in a patient with Niemann-Pick disease. The white-gray appearance of retina is due to diffuse infiltration of ganglion cells with sphingomyelin. The dark red appearance of the fovea is due to the transmission of choroidal color through the relatively thin retina in the central foveal region.

20 Angioid Streaks

Angioid streaks are irregular "spoke-like" reddish brown bands located deep to the retina that appear to radiate from the optic disc (**Figs. 20.1 and 20.2**). They represent cracks in Bruch's membrane. Visual loss may occur when the streaks involve the fovea or when choroidal neovascularization and hemorrhage develop.

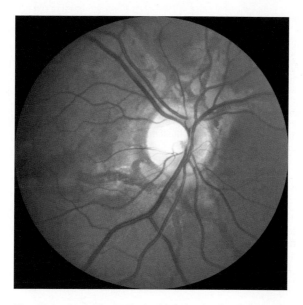

Fig. 20.1 Angioid streaks—reddish brown bands, located deep to the retina, surrounding the optic disc and radiating from it in an irregular "spoke-like" pattern.

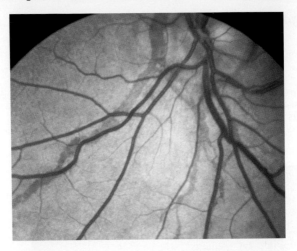

Fig. 20.2   Angioid streaks—dark red bands, located deep to the retina, radiating away from the optic disc. The lesions are at the level of Bruch's membrane. Retinal vessels are seen crossing over these lesions.

Conditions Associated with Angioid Streaks

- Idiopathic (50%)
- Pseudoxanthoma elasticum
- Ehlers-Danlos syndrome
- Sickle cell disease
- Paget disease
- Marfan syndrome
- Acromegaly
- Lead poisoning

21 Optic Disc Swelling

Optic disc swelling is abnormal elevation of the optic disc with blurring of its margins. The term *papilledema* is used to describe swelling of the optic disc secondary to the elevation of intracranial pressure.

Differential Diagnosis

◆ Papilledema (**Fig. 21.1**)
◆ Anterior optic neuritis (papillitis)
◆ Central retinal vein occlusion
◆ Anterior ischemic optic neuropathy
◆ Toxic optic neuropathy
◆ Hereditary optic neuropathy
◆ Neuroretinitis
◆ Diabetic papillopathy
◆ Hypertension (**Fig. 21.2**)
◆ Respiratory failure
◆ Carotid-cavernous fistula
◆ Optic disc/nerve infiltration
  ◦ Tumors of the optic nerve—glioma
  ◦ Lymphoma
  ◦ Leukemia
  ◦ Sarcoidosis
  ◦ Granulomatous infections
◆ Ocular conditions
  ◦ Ocular hypotony
  ◦ Chronic intraocular inflammation
  ◦ Optic disc drusen—pseudopapilledema
  ◦ High hypermetropia—pseudopapilledema

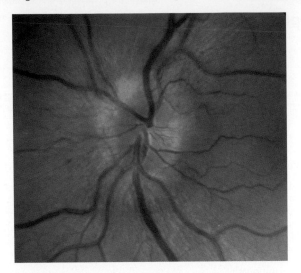

Fig. 21.1 Optic disc swelling with blurring of the margins in a patient with early-stage papilledema and idiopathic intracranial hypertension.

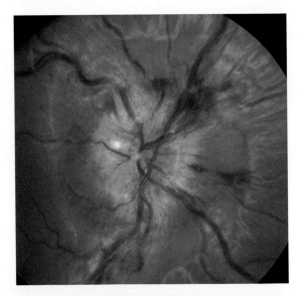

Fig. 21.2 Optic disc swelling, blurring of the margins, retinal folds, and hemorrhages in a patient with severe ("malignant") systemic hypertension.

22 Choroidal Folds

Choroidal folds often appear as horizontally oriented dark and light striae that most commonly involve the macular region (**Fig. 22.1**). Choroidal folds that occur in the fundus periphery (e.g., after a resolved choroidal detachment) are often curvilinear.

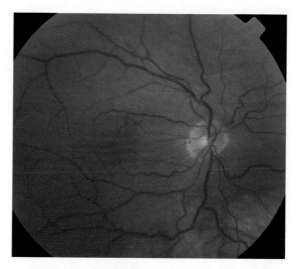

Fig. 22.1 Choroidal folds—horizontally oriented dark and light stripes at the macular region due to choroidal folds.

Conditions Associated with Choroidal Folds

◆ Thyroid eye disease
◆ Orbital mass
◆ Orbital inflammation
◆ Posterior scleritis
◆ Intraocular mass
◆ Papilledema
◆ Epiretinal membrane—usually cause retinal folds rather than "true" choroidal/retinal pigment epithelium (RPE) folds (**Fig. 22.2**)
◆ Ocular hypotony
◆ Resolved choroidal detachment
◆ Scleral surgery
◆ Choroidal neovascularization
◆ Severe hyperopia
◆ Nanophthalmos
◆ Drugs—sulfa antibiotics, acetazolamide, hydrochlorothiazide, metronidazole
◆ Idiopathic

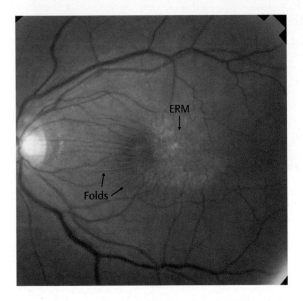

Fig. 22.2   Contraction of epiretinal membrane (ERM) resulting in distortion of the vitreomacular interface with horizontal and radial folds of the retinal surface.

Bone-Spicule Pigmentation

◆ Retinitis pigmentosa and its variants (**Fig. 23.1**)
◆ Pigmentary retinopathy in systemic diseases
  ◦ Usher syndrome
  ◦ Abetalipoproteinemia
  ◦ Refsum disease
  ◦ Kearns-Sayre syndrome
  ◦ Alström syndrome
  ◦ Cockayne syndrome
  ◦ Friedreich ataxia
  ◦ Mucopolysaccharidoses
  ◦ Paraneoplastic syndrome
◆ Age-related reticular pigmentary degeneration
◆ Congenital rubella (salt and pepper retinopathy)
◆ Congenital syphilis
◆ Choroidal ischemia, late stages
◆ Resolved choroidal/retinal detachment

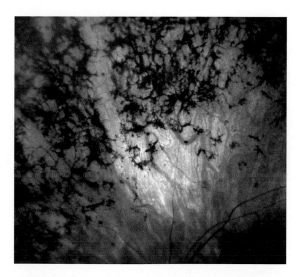

Fig. 23.1 Extensive "bone-spicule" pigmentation in a patient with retinitis pigmentosa.

Flat Pigmented Lesions

◆ Chorioretinal scars
  ◦ Infections
    ◆ Toxoplasma (**Fig. 23.2**)
    ◆ Syphilis
    ◆ Cytomegalovirus
    ◆ Herpes zoster and herpes simplex virus
    ◆ West Nile virus
    ◆ Histoplasmosis (**Fig. 23.3**)
    ◆ Parasitic
    ◆ Bacteremia, fungemia
  ◦ Choroiditis
    ◆ Sarcoidosis
    ◆ Sympathetic ophthalmia
    ◆ Bird-shot choroiditis
    ◆ Vogt-Koyanagi-Harada syndrome
    ◆ Serpiginous choroidopathy
  ◦ Trauma
  ◦ Cryotherapy/laser photocoagulation
  ◦ Age-related macular degeneration
  ◦ Choroidal infarct
    ◆ Severe hypertension
    ◆ Sickle cell hemoglobinopathies
◆ Retinal dystrophies
◆ Choroidal nevus (**Fig. 23.4**)
◆ Congenital hypertrophy of the retinal pigment epithelium (CHRPE) (**Figs. 23.5 and 23.6**)
◆ Drugs
  ◦ Chloroquine/hydroxychloroquine
  ◦ Thioridazine
  ◦ Chlorpromazine
  ◦ Desferrioxamine

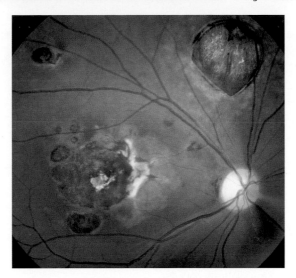

Fig. 23.2   Flat, pigmented lesions due to chorioretinal scarring caused by congenital toxoplasmosis.

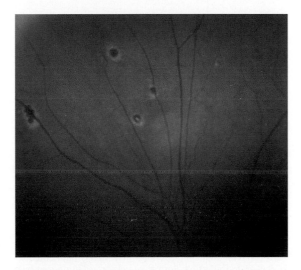

Fig. 23.3   Multiple, focal, pigmented, peripheral chorioretinal scars in a patient with ocular histoplasmosis syndrome.

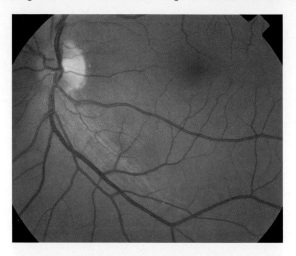

Fig. 23.4 Asymptomatic, pigmented, flat choroidal nevus inferotemporal to the optic disc.

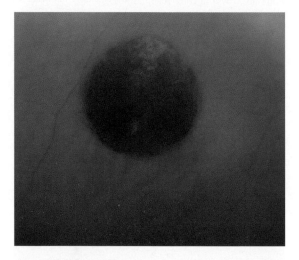

Fig. 23.5 Congenital hypertrophy of retinal pigment epithelium (CHRPE)—well circumscribed, flat, darkly pigmented lesion deep to the retina. Retinal vessels are seen passing over the lesion.

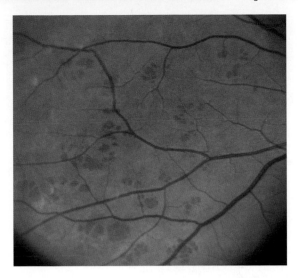

Fig. 23.6 "Bear-tracks" are congenital, small, idiopathic, pigmented lesions in retinal pigment epithelium that occur in groups. The lesions are benign and nonprogressive.

24 Chorioretinal Mass Lesions

◆ Pigmented Lesions

- ◆ Choroidal nevus (usually a flat lesion)
- ◆ Choroidal malignant melanoma (**Fig. 24.1**)
- ◆ Melanocytoma

◆ Nonpigmented Lesions

- ◆ Amelanotic choroidal melanoma
- ◆ Choroidal metastasis (**Fig. 24.2**)
- ◆ Retinoblastoma
- ◆ Granuloma (e.g., toxocara canis) (**Fig. 24.3**)
- ◆ Posterior scleritis
- ◆ Capillary hemangioma
- ◆ Choroidal detachment (may be brown or gray)
- ◆ Choroidal hemorrhage (**Fig. 24.4**)
- ◆ Exudative (wet) age-related macular degeneration (**Fig. 24.5**)
- ◆ Other tumors—osteoma, astrocytoma (e.g., tuberous sclerosis), adenoma of the retinal pigment epithelium (may contain pigment), combined hamartoma of the retina and retinal pigment epithelium, neurilemmoma, leiomyoma

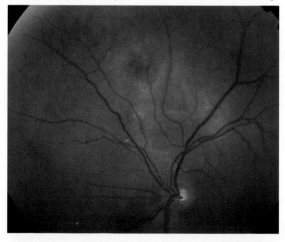

Fig. 24.1 Choroidal malignant melanoma—large pigmented choroidal mass. Overlying "orange" pigment is suggestive of choroidal melanoma.

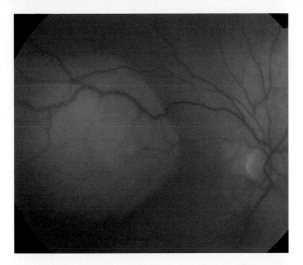

Fig. 24.2 Choroidal metastasis—lightly pigmented choroidal mass.

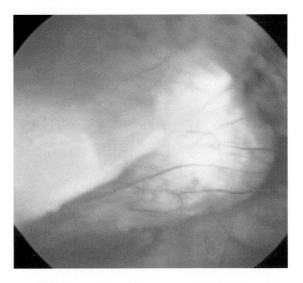

Fig. 24.3 Toxocara granuloma–gray-white lesion with vitreous band in the peripheral fundus caused by toxocara canis.

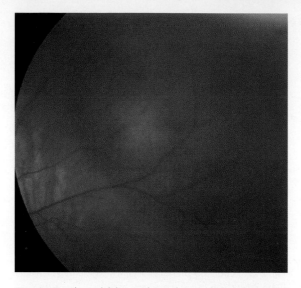

Fig. 24.4 Choroidal hemorrhage—brown/dark red elevated subretinal lesion in a highly myopic patient. The hemorrhage was noted after cataract surgery and resolved within 2 months.

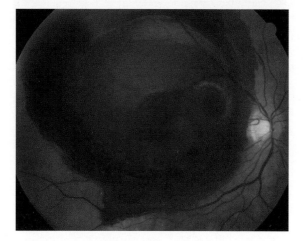

Fig. 24.5 Large area of thick subretinal hemorrhage resembling a pigmented choroidal mass in a patient with exudative "wet" macular degeneration.

25 Vitreous Opacities

In young individuals, the vitreous gel is normally optically clear. Vitreous opacities develop as a result of normal physiologic aging changes (syneresis or liquefaction), or as a result of pathologic processes.

Differential Diagnosis

- Vitreous degeneration—mild opacities
- Vitritis—inflammatory cells within the vitreous (seen on biomicroscopy)
- Vitreous hemorrhage
  - Loculated, fresh—red (**Fig. 25.1**)
  - Diffuse—red haze
  - Old organized—yellow/brown/gray appearance (**Fig. 25.2**)
- Asteroid hyalosis (**Figs. 25.3 and 25.4**)
- Endophthalmitis
- Pigment—trauma, retinal detachment, tumors
- Lymphoma masquerading as vitritis
- Amyloidosis—"glass wool" vitreous veils/clouds
- Cholesterolosis
- Lens material
  - Dislocated crystalline lens
  - Retained lens material after cataract surgery
- Foreign body
- Cysticercosis
- Whipple disease
- Developmental cysts
- Iatrogenic
  - Intravitreal drugs (e.g., triamcinolone acetonide)
  - Intravitreal gas (e.g., surgery for retinal detachment)

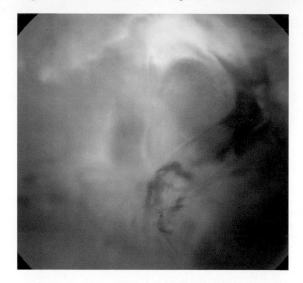

Fig. 25.1 Vitreous opacities due to old (yellow-white) and recent (red) vitreous hemorrhage in a patient with proliferative diabetic retinopathy.

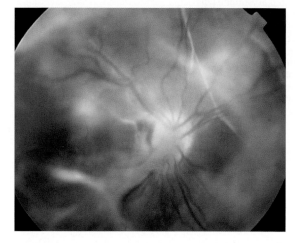

Fig. 25.2 Yellow-white vitreous opacities due to long-standing traumatic vitreous hemorrhage. Subretinal bands are also present.

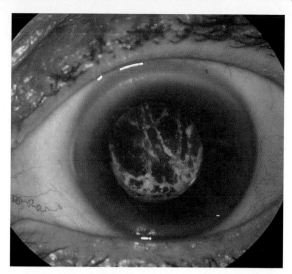

Fig. 25.3 Asteroid hyalosis—strings of whitish refractile particles in the vitreous cavity seen within the pupil in this patient with diabetes. If a cataract is present, the opacities usually are yellow in appearance.

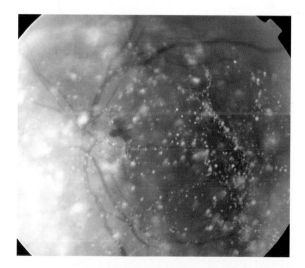

Fig. 25.4 Asteroid hyalosis—multiple whitish refractile particles in the vitreous cavity obscuring the view of the fundus in a patient with diabetic retinopathy.

III
The Retina in Systemic Disease

◆ Diabetic Retinopathy

Diabetic retinopathy is the most common cause of blindness in the working-age population. The occurrence of diabetic retinopathy is associated with duration of diabetes, poor glycemic control, hypertension, diabetic nephropathy, pregnancy, and smoking. Approximately 25% of all diabetics have some form of diabetic retinopathy. After 20 years of diabetes, retinopathy occurs in over 95% of individuals with type 1 and 60% of individuals with type 2 diabetes; approximately 3% of patients with type 1 diabetes become legally blind after 20 years.

Pathophysiology (Fig. 26.1)

Diabetic retinopathy is a microvasculopathy that causes microvascular occlusion and leakage. An early effect of diabetic retinopathy is breakdown of the blood–retinal barrier.

Microvascular occlusion is caused by the following:
◆ Thickening of capillary basement membrane
◆ Abnormal proliferation of capillary endothelium
◆ Increased platelet adhesion
◆ Increased blood viscosity
◆ Defective fibrinolysis

Microvascular leakage is caused by the following:
◆ Impairment of endothelial tight junctions
◆ Loss of pericytes
◆ Weakening of capillary wall
◆ Elevated levels of vascular endothelial growth factor (VEGF)—Abnormally elevated VEGF levels result in increased vascular permeability and angiogenesis manifesting as retinal edema and neovascularization.

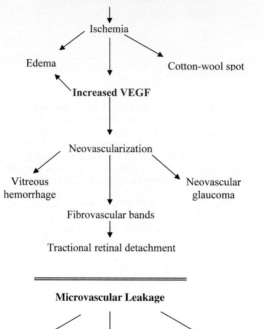

Fig. 26.1 Microvascular occlusion and leakage. VEGF, vascular endothelial growth factor.

Symptoms

◆ Visually asymptomatic—Most patients with early diabetic retinopathy are visually asymptomatic.
◆ Transient, fluctuating blurring of vision—associated with fluctuations in blood glucose levels affecting the lens or the retina
◆ Gradual loss of vision
  ◦ Macular edema
  ◦ Tractional retinal detachment
  ◦ Cataract
◆ Acute loss of vision
  ◦ Vitreous hemorrhage
  ◦ Retinal vascular occlusion
  ◦ Rhegmatogenous or tractional retinal detachment
◆ Floaters
  ◦ Vitreous syneresis
  ◦ Vitreous detachment
  ◦ Vitreous hemorrhage
◆ Pain
  ◦ Neovascular glaucoma
  ◦ Corneal epithelial erosions

Fundus Features

◆ Retinal hemorrhages
  ◦ Superficial flame-shaped hemorrhages (**Fig. 26.2**)
  ◦ Dot hemorrhages
  ◦ Blot hemorrhages (**Fig. 26.3**)
  ◦ Preretinal hemorrhages
  ◦ Subhyaloid hemorrhages (**Fig. 26.4**)
◆ Microaneurysms—small, round, red dots, 10 to 50 μm in diameter, located within the retina
◆ Retinal edema—focal or diffuse areas of retinal thickening with blunted light reflex
◆ Hard exudates—well-circumscribed, shiny, yellow intraretinal deposits represent chronic capillary leakage (**Fig. 26.5**)
◆ Cotton-wool spots (CWSs)—small, yellow-white, superficial, feathery lesions; represent impairment of axonal transport due to focal ischemia
◆ Venous beading—irregular caliber of veins (**Fig. 26.6**)
◆ Venous loops (**Fig. 26.7**)
◆ Intraretinal microvascular abnormalities (IRMAs)
◆ Neovascularization at the optic disc (NVD)
◆ Neovascularization elsewhere in the retina (NVE)
◆ Vitreous hemorrhage
◆ Macular folds
◆ Tractional retinal detachment (TDR)
◆ Combined tractional/rhegmatogenous retinal detachment

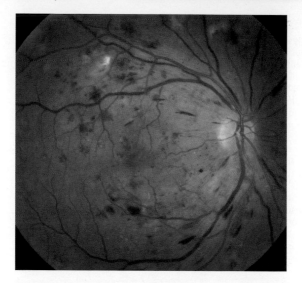

Fig. 26.2 Superficial, flame-shaped retinal hemorrhages, dot hemorrhages, microaneurysms, and cotton-wool spots in a patient with severe nonproliferative diabetic retinopathy.

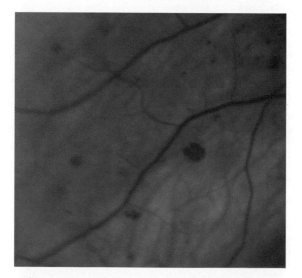

Fig. 26.3 Dot and blot hemorrhages in a patient with nonproliferative diabetic retinopathy. Blot hemorrhages are larger and darker than dot hemorrhages and are located in deeper layers of the retina.

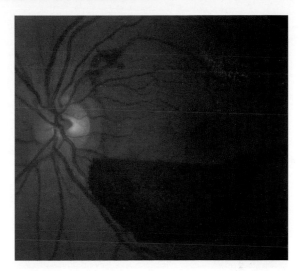

Fig. 26.4 Subhyaloid hemorrhage from retinal neovascularization in proliferative diabetic retinopathy. Subhyaloid hemorrhage is located within the space between the inner surface of the retina and the posterior hyaloid face. The upper border is usually straight with a "fluid level"; it obscures the retinal blood vessels, which run posterior (external) to it.

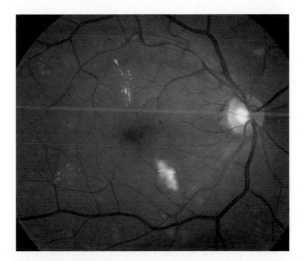

Fig. 26.5 Cotton-wool spots, hard exudates, microaneurysms, and small hemorrhages in a patient with poorly controlled diabetes.

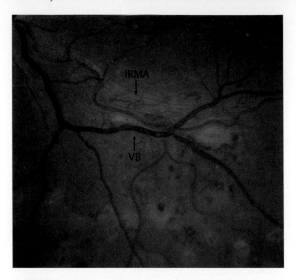

Fig. 26.6 Venous beading (VB) and intraretinal microvascular abnormalities (IRMAs) in a patient with treated proliferative diabetic retinopathy. Panretinal laser photocoagulation scars are present in the lower part of the photograph.

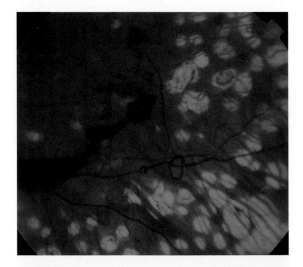

Fig. 26.7 Vascular loops, preretinal and intraretinal hemorrhages, and scars of panretinal laser photocoagulation in a patient with proliferative diabetic retinopathy (PDR).

Classification of Diabetic Retinopathy

There are four main categories of diabetic retinopathy:

◆ Nonproliferative diabetic retinopathy (NPDR)
◆ Proliferative diabetic retinopathy (PDR)
◆ Diabetic macular edema (DME)
◆ Ischemic maculopathy

Diabetic macular edema and ischemic maculopathy may coexist and can occur in conjunction with PDR as well as NPDR.

Nonproliferative Diabetic Retinopathy

NPDR is retinopathy in the absence of retinal and optic disc neovascularization. It includes dot and blot and superficial hemorrhages, microaneurysms, hard exudates, CWSs, venous beading, venous loops, and IRMAs. NPDR is further classified into mild, moderate, and severe (**Figs. 26.8, 26.9, and 26.10**).

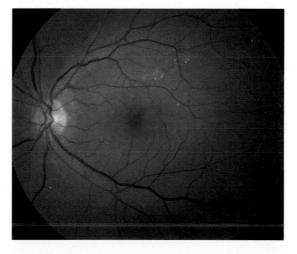

Fig. 26.8   Microaneurysms, fine hard exudates, and dot hemorrhages in a patient with mild nonproliferative diabetic retinopathy (background diabetic retinopathy).

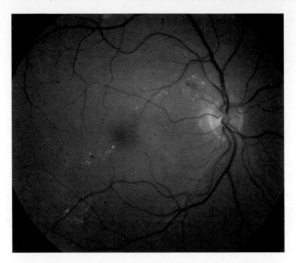

Fig. 26.9 Moderate nonproliferative diabetic retinopathy–multiple microaneurysms, small hemorrhages, and fine hard exudates are present.

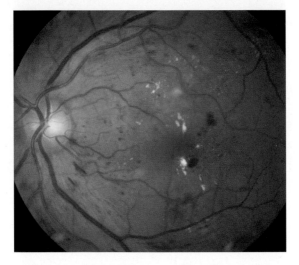

Fig. 26.10 Severe nonproliferative diabetic retinopathy with clinically significant macular edema. Extensive hemorrhages and cotton-wool spots are present. Hard exudates are encroaching on the fovea.

Preproliferative diabetic retinopathy (severe NPDR) is characterized by severe ischemia, but absence of neovascularization. Patients with preproliferative diabetic retinopathy are at high risk of developing neovascularization (15% within 1 year). Retinal signs indicative of ischemia include severe intraretinal hemorrhages in all retinal quadrants, venous beading, IRMA, and multiple CWSs (**Figs. 26.11 and 26.12**).

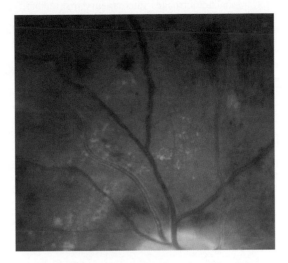

Fig. 26.11 Severe nonproliferative diabetic retinopathy. Venous beading (irregular caliber), multiple hemorrhages, and hard exudates are present.

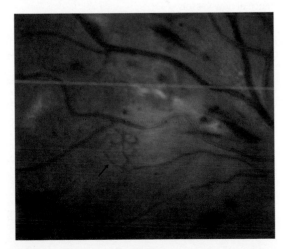

Fig. 26.12 Severe nonproliferative diabetic retinopathy— IRMAs (*arrow*), multiple hemorrhages, and cotton-wool spots.

Table 26.1 lists the stages of NPDR.

Table 26.1　Stages of Nonproliferative Diabetic Retinopathy (NPDR)

◆ Mild NPDR—background diabetic retinopathy (BGDR)
　◦ Few intraretinal hemorrhages, microaneurysms, and hard exudates
◆ Moderate NPDR
　◦ Moderate intraretinal hemorrhages, microaneurysms, and hard exudates
◆ Severe NPDR—4:2:1 rule
　◦ Intraretinal hemorrhages and microaneurysms in four quadrants
　◦ Venous beading in two or more quadrants
　◦ Intraretinal microvascular abnormalities in one or more quadrants

Proliferative Diabetic Retinopathy

PDR is characterized by the development of NVD or NVE (**Table 26.2, Figs. 26.13, 26.14, and 26.15**). PDR is considered non–high-risk when NVD or NVE are extremely small and there is no vitreous hemorrhage (**Fig. 26.16**). But PDR is high-risk when the NVD is larger than one fourth of the disc area, or when NVE and vitreous hemorrhage are present (**Figs. 26.17 and 26.18**). High-risk PDR warrants prompt panretinal laser photocoagulation, whereas non–high-risk PDR may be closely observed until signs of progression occur.

Table 26.2　Characteristics of High-Risk Proliferative Diabetic Retinopathy (PDR)

Any combination of three of the following four findings:
◆ Presence of new vessels
◆ New vessels on the surface of the optic disc or within 1 disc diameter of the disc (NVD)
◆ Moderate to severe extent of new vessels; i.e., greater than one fourth of the disc area for NVD, and greater than half a disc area for NVE
◆ Presence of vitreous or preretinal hemorrhage

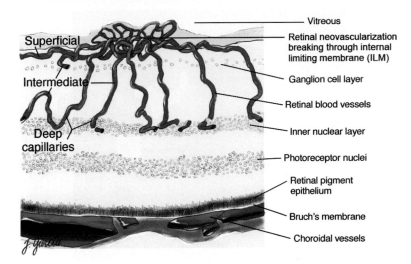

Vitreous

Retinal neovascularization breaking through internal limiting membrane (ILM)

Superficial

Intermediate

Ganglion cell layer

Retinal blood vessels

Deep capillaries

Inner nuclear layer

Photoreceptor nuclei

Retinal pigment epithelium

Bruch's membrane

Choroidal vessels

Fig. 26.13 Neovascular (NV) complexes arise from the superficial and deep retinal vascular networks. NV complexes grow through the internal limiting membrane and into the vitreous cavity or may spread over the retinal surface. (Drawing by Juan R. Garcia. Used with permission of Johns Hopkins University.)

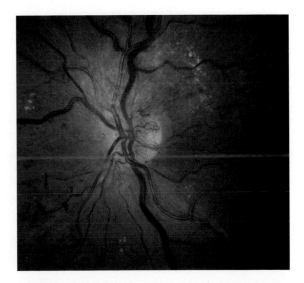

Fig. 26.14 Neovascularization at the optic disc (NVD). Fronds of new vessels cover approximately half of the optic disc area. IRMAs are present (*arrow*).

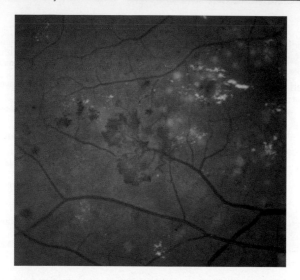

Fig. 26.15 Neovascularization elsewhere (NVE)—neovascular complex in the inferotemporal part of the right macula in a patient with proliferative diabetic retinopathy.

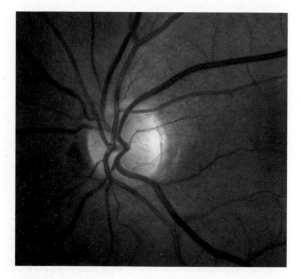

Fig. 26.16 Early neovascularization at the optic disc (NVD)—fine fronds of new vessels covering less than one fourth of the optic disc area.

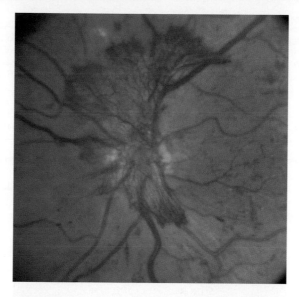

Fig. 26.17 Extensive neovascular fronds arising from the optic disc (NVD) and extending to the surrounding retina and into the vitreous cavity. This patient has a high risk for vitreous hemorrhage.

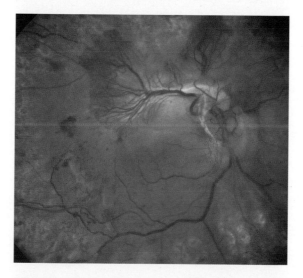

Fig. 26.18 Extensive fibrovascular proliferation involving the optic disc and the superior vascular arcade. Early tractional retinal detachment and prior retinal laser photocoagulation scars are present.

Diabetic Macular Edema

Diabetic macular edema may manifest as focal or diffuse retinal thickening with or without the presence of hard exudates. It may occur in conjunction with NPDR or PDR. The term *clinically significant macular edema* (CSME) is used when retinal edema extends to or threatens the fovea (**Table 26.3**) (**Figs. 26.19, 26.20, 26.21, and 26.22**). The visual acuity may or may not be affected.

Table 26.3   Characteristics of Clinically Significant Macular Edema (CSME)

◆ Thickening of retina within 500 μm of the foveal center
◆ Hard exudates within 500 μm of the foveal center if associated with thickening of the adjacent retina
◆ Area of retinal thickening 1 disc diameter or larger within 1 disc diameter of the foveal center

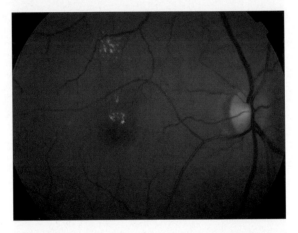

Fig. 26.19   Clinically significant macular edema (CSME). Hard exudates are present within 500 μm of the foveal center.

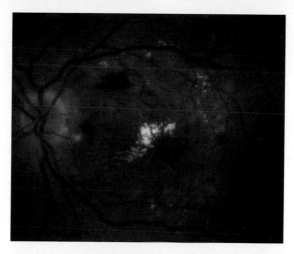

Fig. 26.20 Clinically significant macular edema (CSME)—plaques of hard exudates involving the foveal region. Scars of prior focal laser photocoagulation are present.

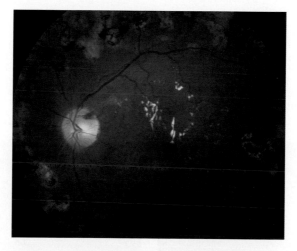

Fig. 26.21 Clinically significant macular edema (CSME). Hard exudates are present in a circinate pattern superior to the fovea in this patient with a history of proliferative diabetic retinopathy and macular edema. Panretinal laser photocoagulation scars are present.

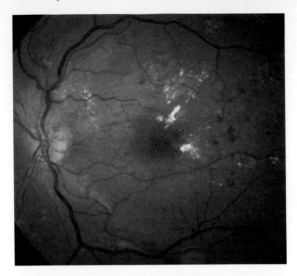

Fig. 26.22 Neovascularization at the disc (NVD), hemorrhages, and hard exudates in a patient with PDR and clinically significant macular edema.

Ischemic Maculopathy

Ischemic maculopathy is characterized by a varying degree of macular edema and evidence of capillary nonperfusion on fluorescein angiography (**Fig. 26.23**). The visual acuity is usually diminished. Ischemic maculopathy may occur in conjunction with NPDR or PDR. Ischemic maculopathy responds less favorably to treatment than macular edema without ischemia.

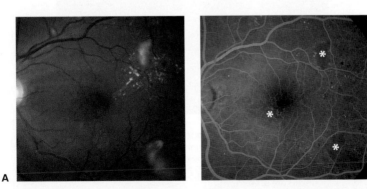

Fig. 26.23 Ischemic macular edema. **(A)** Color photograph showing hard exudates extending to the vicinity of the fovea, and telangiectasis inferior and nasal to the fovea in this patient with diabetic maculopathy. **(B)** Fundus fluorescein angiogram showing areas of capillary nonperfusion (*asterisks*).

Advanced Diabetic Eye Disease

Advanced diabetic eye disease arises as the result of progressive fibrovascular proliferation.

- ◆ Vitreous hemorrhage (**Figs. 26.24 and 26.25**)
- ◆ TRD—caused by the contraction of fibrovascular bands that exert traction on the retina (**Fig. 26.26 and 26.27**)
- ◆ Combined tractional-rhegmatogenous retinal detachment (CTRRD)—is caused when progressive, severe traction results in formation of retinal breaks (**Fig. 26.28**)
- ◆ Neovascularization of iris/neovascular glaucoma (**Fig. 26.29**)

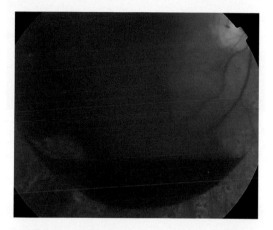

Fig. 26.24 Vitreous hemorrhage—large subhyaloid hemorrhage with red blood cells gravitating inferiorly, resulting in a "fluid level." Scars of prior panretinal laser photocoagulation are present.

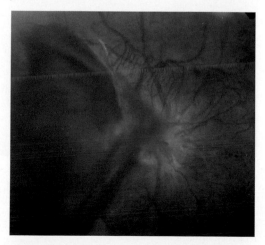

Fig. 26.25 Severe neovascularization at the optic disc and surrounding retina, with overlying vitreous hemorrhage, in a patient with proliferative diabetic retinopathy.

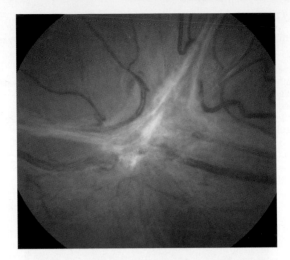

Fig. 26.26 Localized tractional retinal detachment (TRD). Contraction of fibroproliferative tissue has resulted in vitreoretinal traction, causing distortion of the blood vessels and localized elevation of the retina.

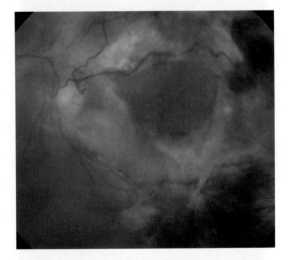

Fig. 26.27 Severe fibrovascular proliferation and tractional retinal detachment (TRD). Contraction of fibrovascular membranes has resulted in severe TRD. Localized areas of vitreous hemorrhage are present adjacent to neovascular complexes. The view of the fundus is hazy due to diffuse vitreous hemorrhage.

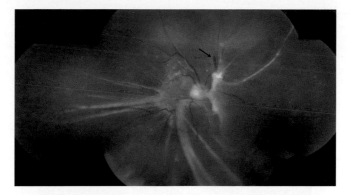

Fig. 26.28 Combined tractional-rhegmatogenous retinal detachment (CTRRD)—total retinal detachment with multiple folds and contracted posterior hyaloid with fibroproliferative tissue. A posterior, slit-like, paravascular retinal tear (*arrow*), typically seen in diabetic CTRRD, is present superonasal to the optic disc.

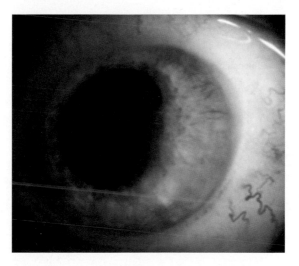

Fig. 26.29 Neovascularization of iris (rubeosis). Invasion of the angle with fronds of new vessels has resulted in neovascular glaucoma, which has caused the cornea to be edematous and hazy.

Diabetic Papillopathy

Diabetic papillopathy is typically a self-limiting condition presenting with unilateral or bilateral moderate visual loss and swelling of the optic disc in the presence of diabetic retinopathy (**Fig. 26.30**). Spontaneous resolution and improvement of vision often occurs over a period of weeks.

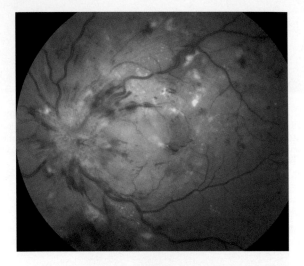

Fig. 26.30   Diabetic papillopathy. The optic disc is swollen and hyperemic. Peripapillary hemorrhages and extensive signs of diabetic retinopathy are present.

Management

General

◆ Blood glucose control
◆ Blood pressure control
◆ Serum lipid management
◆ Health education, weight management, cessation of smoking, exercise

Fundus Examination

Annual dilated fundus examination is recommended for all patients with diabetes and no evidence of diabetic retinopathy. Patients with diabetic retinopathy require more frequent examinations, depending on the type and severity of retinopathy.

Clinically Significant Macular Edema

◆ Focal laser photocoagulation (**Figs. 26.31 and 26.32**)
◆ Intravitreal corticosteroid injection
  ◦ Triamcinolone acetonide (Kenalog; currently under investigation)
◆ Intravitreal anti-VEGF injection (currently under investigation)
  ◦ Bevacizumab (Avastin)
  ◦ Ranibizumab (Lucentis)

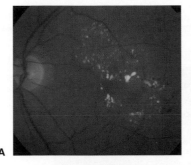 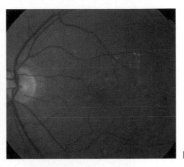

A **B**

Fig. 26.31 **(A)** Clinically significant macular edema (CSME) in a patient with nonproliferative diabetic retinopathy prior to treatment with focal laser photocoagulation. **(B)** Resolution of hard exudates 6 months after focal laser photocoagulation. Faint photocoagulation scars are present.

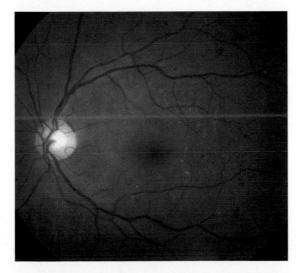

Fig. 26.32 Focal laser photocoagulation scars in a patient who was treated for clinically significant macular edema. Minor residual hard exudates are present.

Proliferative Diabetic Retinopathy

◆ Non–high-risk
  ◦ Regular monitoring by retinal specialist
  ◦ Panretinal laser photocoagulation (PRP) may be considered in patients with poor compliance with follow-up, and in those with additional risk factors, such as poorly controlled diabetes, severe hypertension, renal failure, pregnancy, and aggressive proliferative disease in the fellow eye.
◆ High-risk
  ◦ Prompt PRP (**Fig. 26.33, 26.34, and 26.35**)
  ◦ Intravitreal anti-VEGF injections can be useful adjunctive therapy when concurrent vitreous hemorrhage prevents effective laser applications (currently under investigation).

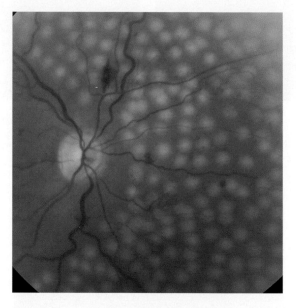

Fig. 26.33   Panretinal laser photocoagulation (PRP)—multiple yellow-white laser marks 30 minutes after PRP.

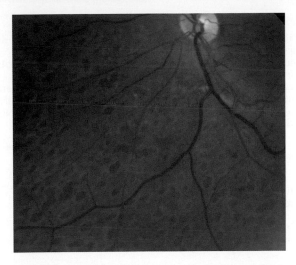

Fig. 26.34 Panretinal laser photocoagulation (PRP)—multiple focal pigmented chorioretinal scars 3 months after PRP.

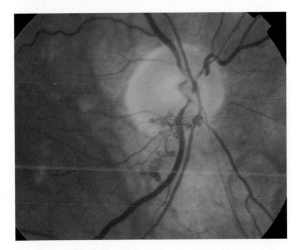

Fig. 26.35 Regressed neovascularization at the disc (NVD). The vascular meshwork consists of larger caliber vessels and has lost its fine fronds at its margins, compared with active new vessel complexes.

Vitreous Hemorrhage

◆ PRP (if the vitreous hemorrhage clears or is mild enough to allow delivery of laser photocoagulation)

◆ Vitrectomy and endolaser photocoagulation if the vitreous hemorrhage does not clear spontaneously over one to several months

◆ Treatment with intravitreal anti-VEGF medications may be considered to stabilize the neovascular process while the vitreous hemorrhage clears, thereby allowing delivery of PRP. Preoperative administration of anti-VEGF agents may reduce the risk of intraoperative hemorrhage.

Neovascular Glaucoma

◆ Medications for lowering intraocular pressure

◆ Intravitreal anti-VEGF medications (currently under investigation)

◆ PRP

◆ Glaucoma surgery

◆ Vitrectomy and endolaser photocoagulation

Retinal Detachment

◆ Retinal detachment surgery, including vitrectomy, removal of fibroproliferative tissue, and panretinal endolaser photocoagulation

Differential Diagnosis of Diabetic Retinopathy

◆ Hypertensive retinopathy

◆ Central or branch retinal vein occlusion—usually unilateral

◆ Carotid artery disease

◆ Sickle cell retinopathy

◆ Radiation retinopathy

◆ Vasculitis

◆ HIV retinopathy

◆ Neuroretinitis

◆ Purtscher-like retinopathy

◆ Other forms of retinal vasculopathy (see Chapters 6, 7, 9, and 11 for the differential diagnosis of retinal hemorrhages, hard exudates, cotton-wool spots, and retinal neovascularization).

◆ Thyroid Disorders

Thyroid eye disease primarily manifests in the orbit, external eye, and the eyelids. The basic pathophysiologic processes include chronic inflammatory infiltration, edema, and deposition of mucopolysaccharides within the orbital fat and extraocular muscles. Later stages of the disease are characterized by fibrosis of the orbital tissues and extraocular muscles. The fundus findings are usually secondary to the presence of orbital disease and include retinal and choroidal folds, optic disc swelling, and optic atrophy.

Symptoms

◆ Dry-eye symptoms/foreign body sensation
◆ Change in appearance of eyes/prominent eyes
◆ Lid swelling
◆ Blurred vision
◆ Diplopia

Fundus Features

◆ Chorioretinal folds (**Fig. 26.36**)—Chorioretinal folds develop as a result of distortion of the posterior wall of the globe by an increased orbital mass effect.
◆ Optic disc swelling—Optic disc swelling develops due to compression of the optic nerve, resulting in impaired axoplasmic flow and reduced venous outflow.
◆ Optic atrophy—due to chronic compression of the optic nerve

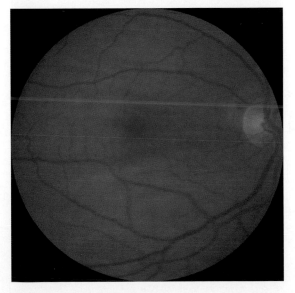

Fig. 26.36 Macular folds in a patient with severe thyroid orbitopathy.

Other Ophthalmic Features

◆ Lid retraction (**Fig. 26.37**)
◆ Lid lag
◆ Conjunctival/episcleral hyperemia—particularly over the extraocular muscle insertions
◆ Chemosis
◆ Superior limbic keratoconjunctivitis
◆ Corneal exposure
◆ Corneal ulcer
◆ Ocular motility disturbance
◆ Proptosis (exophthalmos)
◆ Optic nerve compression
  ◦ Loss of vision
  ◦ Abnormal color vision
  ◦ Scotoma
  ◦ Relative afferent pupillary defect
  ◦ Optic disc swelling
  ◦ Optic atrophy

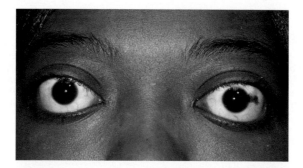

Fig. 26.37   Exophthalmos and eyelid retraction in a patient with thyroid eye disease.

Pearls

• Regular retinal examination is an integral part of the care of the diabetic patient. Initially, some patients may find retinal examination inconvenient and uncomfortable. Explaining the reason for the retinal evaluation and the examination procedure will put the patient at ease, will make the examination easier for the patient and the doctor, and will increase likelihood of compliance with future evaluations.

• The visit for the eye examination can also be used as an opportunity to counsel the patient on risk reduction, including optimal blood glucose and blood pressure control, serum lipid management, and importance of compliance with medications and regular evaluations.

• In situations where diabetic retinopathy has not reached absolute treatment threshold, such as in non–high-risk PDR and borderline CSME, consider the severity of the disease in the fellow eye, and the ability of the patient to comply with regular evaluations.

27 Cardiovascular Disorders

◆ Systemic Hypertension

Effects of Systemic Hypertension on the Eye and Vision

- ◆ Hypertensive retinopathy
- ◆ Hypertensive choroidopathy
- ◆ Hypertensive optic neuropathy
- ◆ Central and branch retinal vein occlusion
- ◆ Retinal macroaneurysm
- ◆ Vitreous hemorrhage
- ◆ Subconjunctival hemorrhage
- ◆ Secondary effects
  - ○ Carotid disease—retinal arterial emboli
  - ○ Cerebrovascular accident—visual field loss
  - ○ Ischemic optic neuropathy
  - ○ Oculomotor cranial nerve palsies
  - ○ Cataract, glaucoma, age-related macular degeneration

Hypertensive Retinopathy

Hypertensive retinopathy is usually asymptomatic. In severe hypertension, however, painless loss of vision may occur due to the development of vitreous or retinal hemorrhages, retinal edema, retinal vascular occlusion, serous retinal detachment, choroidal ischemia, or optic neuropathy.

Fundus Features

- ◆ Focal or diffuse narrowing of retinal arterioles
- ◆ Increased vascular tortuosity (**Fig. 27.1**)
- ◆ Arteriovenous nicking (nipping) (**Fig. 27.2**)
- ◆ Retinal hemorrhages (**Fig. 27.3**)
  - ○ Flame-shaped hemorrhage
  - ○ Dot and blot hemorrhage
  - ○ Preretinal hemorrhage
- ◆ Microaneurysms
- ◆ Hard exudates, macular star
- ◆ Cotton-wool spots (**Figs. 27.4 and 27.5**)
- ◆ Abnormality of vascular reflex
  - ○ Copper-wire reflex (**Fig. 27.6**)
  - ○ Silver-wire reflex (**Fig. 27.7**)
- ◆ Intraretinal microvascular abnormalities
- ◆ Retinal edema (**Fig. 27.8**)
- ◆ Serous retinal detachment—occurs secondary to hypertensive choroidopathy in patients with very severe hypertension or eclampsia (**Fig. 27.9**)
- ◆ Elschnig spots—small to medium-size hyper- and hypopigmented patches representing chorioretinal scarring due to prior choroidal infarction (**Figs. 27.10 and 27.11**)

◆ Siegrist streaks—linear configurations of hyperpigmentation that have a patho-
   genesis similar to that of Elschnig spots.
◆ Optic disc edema (**Fig. 27.12**)
◆ Optic atrophy
◆ Vitreous hemorrhage

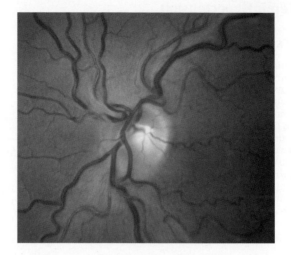

Fig. 27.1   Increased retinal vascular tortuosity in a patient
with chronic systemic hypertension.

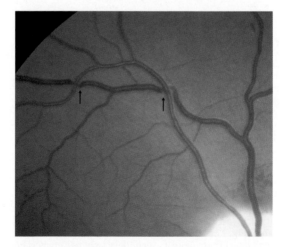

Fig. 27.2   Arteriovenous nicking (*arrows*) is narrowing of the
retinal vein at the site of crossing of an artery. It results from
thickening of the retinal arterial wall in chronic hypertension.

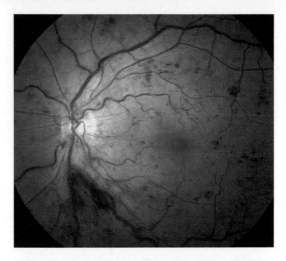

Fig. 27.3   Grade 3 hypertensive retinopathy—multiple dot and blot hemorrhages, flame-shaped hemorrhages, and microaneurysms in a patient with uncontrolled hypertension.

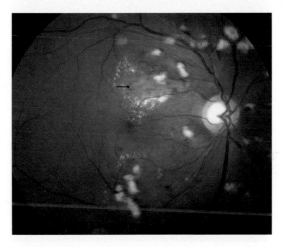

Fig. 27.4   Grade 3 hypertensive retinopathy—multiple flame-shaped hemorrhages, cotton-wool spots, hard exudates, and area of retinal edema (*arrow*).

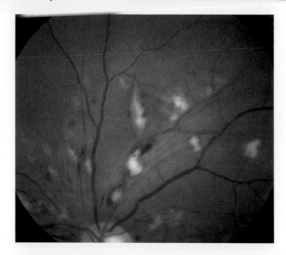

Fig. 27.5 Cotton-wool spots, flame-shaped hemorrhages, and arteriovenous nicking in a patient with hypertension.

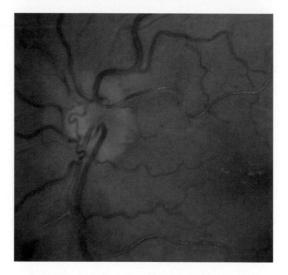

Fig. 27.6 Copper-wire reflex, vascular tortuosity, and blurring of optic disc margin in a patient with severe hypertension.

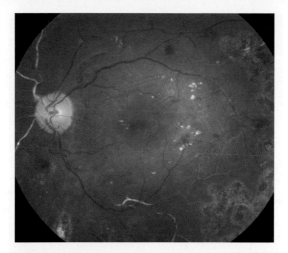

Fig. 27.7 Silver-wire reflex, hard exudates, and hemorrhages are present in a patient with a history of malignant hypertension. Scars of retinal laser photocoagulation are present.

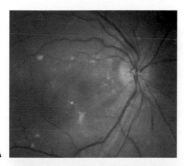

A

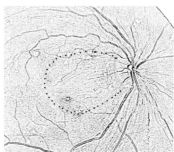

B

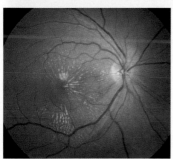

C

Fig. 27.8 **(A)** Retinal edema, multiple cotton-wool spots, and fine hard exudates in a 32-year-old man presenting with blurring of vision and blood pressure of 220/140 mm Hg. **(B)** Area of retinal edema is delineated with dotted line. **(C)** Hard exudates developed in a radial pattern (macular star) 6 weeks after lowering of blood pressure and resolution of the retinal edema.

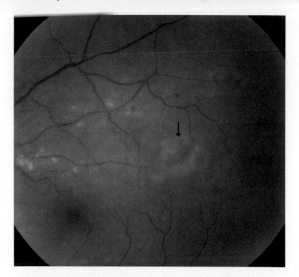

Fig. 27.9 Patchy area of choroidal infarct (*arrow*) with overlying serous retinal detachment in a patient with severe hypertension.

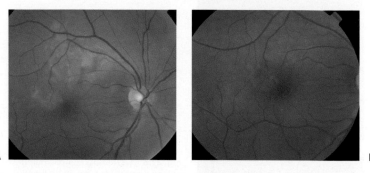

A   B

Fig. 27.10 **(A)** Yellow, placoid, subretinal lesions indicating choroidal ischemia in a patient with severe systemic hypertension. **(B)** Pigmented atrophic scars developed in the areas of choroidal ischemia 2 months after the initial presentation.

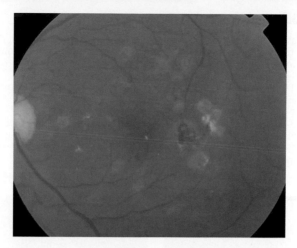

Fig. 27.11 "Elschnig spots"—small to medium-size hyper- and hypopigmented patches representing scarring due to prior hypertension-induced choroidal infarction.

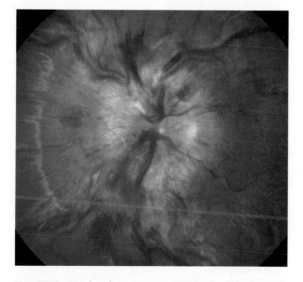

Fig. 27.12 Grade 4 hypertensive retinopathy ("accelerated" or "malignant" hypertension). Optic disc is hyperemic, and edematous with blurring of the margin. Vascular tortuosity and retinal hemorrhages are present.

Classification of Hypertensive Retinopathy

Several classification systems for hypertensive retinopathy have been described, including that by Keith, Wagener, and Barker in 1939. The current conventional classification is:

- Grade 0—no changes
- Grade 1—arteriovenous nicking (nipping), increased vascular tortuosity, and minimal arteriolar narrowing
- Grade 2—arteriolar narrowing with focal irregularities
- Grade 3—retinal hemorrhages, microaneurysms, hard exudates, cotton-wool spots (plus grade 2)
- Grade 4—optic disc swelling (plus grade 3); also termed malignant or accelerated hypertension (**Fig. 27.13**)

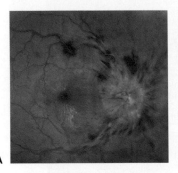 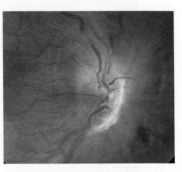

A   B

Fig. 27.13   **(A)** Grade 4 hypertensive retinopathy in a patient with blood pressure of 240/150 mm Hg. Optic disc edema, multiple hemorrhages, and early "macular star" are present. Peripapillary circumferential folds indicate presence of retinal edema and subretinal fluid. **(B)** Prepapillary gliosis, circumferential folds, vascular tortuosity, and hemorrhages 4 months after blood pressure was brought under control.

Differential Diagnosis

- Diabetic retinopathy
- Central or branch retinal vein occlusion
- Papilledema
- Carotid artery disease
- Radiation retinopathy
- Vasculitis
- HIV retinopathy
- Neuroretinitis
- Purtscher-like retinopathy
- Other forms of retinal vasculopathy

◆ Central and Branch Retinal Artery Occlusion (CRAO and BRAO)

Symptoms

- ◆ Acute, painless, monocular loss of vision (rarely bilateral)
  - ◦ Partial (quadrantic or hemifield loss)—branch retinal artery occlusion (BRAO)
  - ◦ Central or paracentral scotoma—small macular branch artery occlusion
  - ◦ Complete—central retinal artery occlusion (CRAO)
  - ◦ Tunnel vision—central retinal artery occlusion with sparing of cilioretinal artery
  - ◦ Transient—amaurosis fugax

Fundus Features

- ◆ Early
  - ◦ Opaque, grayish-white retina (**Fig. 27.14**)
  - ◦ Thickened edematous retina
  - ◦ Obscured retinal pigment epithelium (RPE) and choroidal features (**Fig. 27.15**)
  - ◦ Cherry-red spot at the macula—due to the normally thin anatomy of the retinal layers in the foveal region that allows the reddish light reflex from the intact choroidal vasculature to stand out in contrast to the grayish-white appearance of the surrounding thicker and more opaque retina (**Fig. 27.16**)
  - ◦ Minor retinal hemorrhages
  - ◦ Retinal artery embolus—an embolus is visible in 20 to 30% of cases
  - ◦ Narrow arterioles
  - ◦ Segmented "box-car" arterioles
- ◆ Late
  - ◦ Disappearance of retinal edema and cherry-red spot
  - ◦ Attenuated retinal arterioles
  - ◦ Atrophic, featureless retina
  - ◦ Visible retinal artery embolus
  - ◦ Subtle, diffuse, or patchy pigment mottling
  - ◦ Pale optic disc—optic atrophy
  - ◦ Iris neovascularization—develops in 15% of cases with CRAO. The patient is at highest risk during the first 3 months.

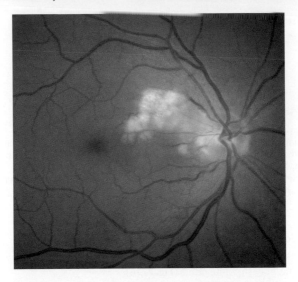

Fig. 27.14 Small branch retinal artery occlusion—yellow-white clouding of retina and cotton-wool spots in the distribution of a small retinal artery. The fovea is spared.

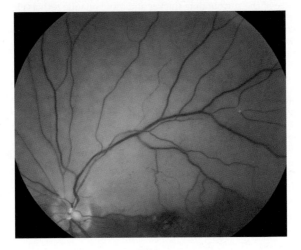

Fig. 27.15 Cloudy swelling of the superior retina in a patient with occlusion of the upper retinal arteries. "Box-carring" of some of the arteries indicates sluggish blood flow. Emboli are visible within the vessels at the optic disc and the superotemporal periphery.

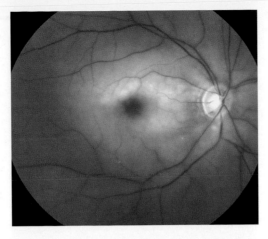

Fig. 27.16 Central retinal artery occlusion. The retina is diffusely edematous and cloudy. "Cherry-red" spot appearance at the macula results from transmission of choroidal color through the relatively thin retina in this region. An embolus is visible in a small retinal arteriole inferior to the fovea.

Causes of Retinal Artery Occlusion

◆ Embolus
  ◦ Platelet emboli (**Fig. 27.17**)—are soft, gray or yellowish, and conform to the shape of the blood vessel. They usually originate from an ulcerating atheromatous plaque within the carotid artery and can cause amaurosis fugax. They may be seen moving along the retinal vasculature.
  ◦ Cholesterol emboli (**Fig. 27.18**)—Hollenhorst plaques are flat, yellow crystalline deposits that are commonly found at the bifurcation of the retinal arteries. They are often asymptomatic. They signify atheromatous disease of the carotid artery.
  ◦ Calcific emboli (**Fig. 27.19 and 27.20**)—Calcific emboli have a pearly white appearance, are larger, and tend to lodge in the larger retinal arteries around the optic disc. Calcific emboli usually occlude the blood flow and are visually symptomatic.
  ◦ Septic emboli—can cause white-centered hemorrhages (Roth spots)
  ◦ Fat emboli—Purtscher-like retinopathy
  ◦ Amniotic fluid emboli—Purtscher-like retinopathy
  ◦ Talc emboli—intravenous drug abuse
◆ Hypercoagulable state
◆ Retinal vasculitis
◆ Sickle cell disease—more frequently affects the smaller peripheral arterioles
◆ Vasospasm—migraine
◆ Dissecting aneurysm of internal carotid artery and its smaller branches
◆ Ocular trauma
◆ Severe elevation of intraocular pressure
  ◦ Acute glaucoma
  ◦ Intraocular surgery
  ◦ External pressure on the eye (e.g., during general anesthesia)
◆ Severe elevation of orbital pressure
  ◦ Acute retrobulbar hemorrhage
◆ Other associations
  ◦ Mitral valve prolapse

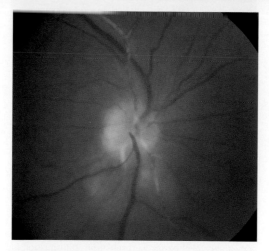

Fig. 27.17 Extensive platelet emboli conforming to the shape of the blood vessels.

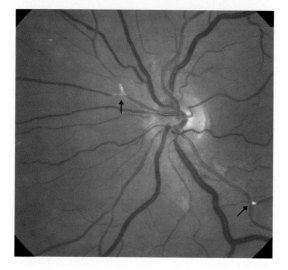

Fig. 27.18 Cholesterol emboli (Hollenhorst plaques) are flat, yellow crystalline deposits that are commonly found at the bifurcation of the retinal arteries (*arrows*). The most common source of this type of embolus is an atheromatous lesion of the carotid artery.

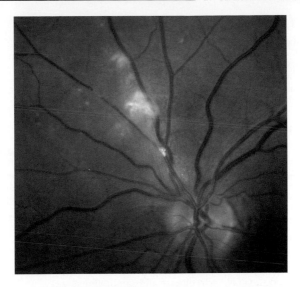

Fig. 27.19 A calcific embolus is impacted at the bifurcation of the superonasal artery. Note attenuation of the artery and dark-colored blood (representing stagnation) distal to the embolus. Cotton-wool spots (CWSs) are present.

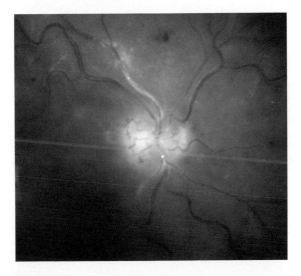

Fig. 27.20 A calcific embolus and platelet emboli are present in the arteries over the optic disc. This patient also had a history of central retinal vein occlusion as evidenced by the collateral vessels on the disc and venous sheathing.

Sources of Retinal Emboli

- Carotid artery atheromatous plaque
- Cardiac valve abnormalities
- Cardiac defects
- Atrial myxoma
- Bacterial endocarditis/septicemia/fungemia
- Intravenous drugs (paradoxical emboli)

Amaurosis Fugax

Amaurosis fugax is due to a transient embolic phenomenon within the retinal circulation, resulting in a transient, monocular, painless loss of vision that usually lasts less than 1 hour. Amaurosis fugax is often associated with other forms of transient ischemic attacks (TIAs) occurring within the carotid artery distribution. During the attack, ophthalmoscopy may show bright yellow cholesterol emboli. The source of these emboli is often carotid atheromatous plaque.

Differential Diagnosis of Cherry-Red Spot in Macula

- Central retinal artery occlusion
- Sphingolipidoses
  - Gangliosidoses (Tay-Sachs disease and Sandhoff disease)
  - Niemann-Pick disease types A to D
  - Metachromatic leukodystrophy
  - Farber disease
- Mucopolysaccharidoses
  - Hurler disease
- Mucolipidoses; sialidoses

Ophthalmic Artery Occlusion

- Severe visual loss, often to the level of light perception or worse. This degree of visual loss is rare in isolated central retinal artery occlusion with retention of choroidal or optic nerve perfusion.
- Pale opaque retina, no cherry-red spot (because choroidal circulation is also diminished)
- Ocular hypotony
- Serous retinal and choroidal detachment
- Bone-spicule pigmentary changes in late stages
- Iris neovascularization

◆ Central and Branch Retinal Vein Occlusion (CRVO and BRVO)

Symptoms

- Acute onset, painless loss of vision corresponding to the area of distribution of the occluded vessel. Loss of vision may not occur in BRVO.

Fundus Features

- Early (**Figs. 27.21 and 27.22**)
  - Superficial retinal hemorrhages—severe cases have a "blood and thunder" appearance
  - Microaneurysms
  - Retinal edema
  - Cotton-wool spots
  - Capillary telangiectasia
  - Blurring of optic disc margin or disc edema
  - Serous retinal detachment—severe cases
- Late (**Figs. 27.23 and 27.24**)
  - Above signs
  - Hard exudates
  - Collateral (shunt) vessels at the optic disc (**Fig. 27.25**)
  - Venous sheathing
  - Retinal or optic disc neovascularization
  - Vitreous hemorrhage
  - Tractional retinal detachment
  - Iris neovascularization—more common in CRVO than in BRVO or CRAO; most cases occur within the first 3 months

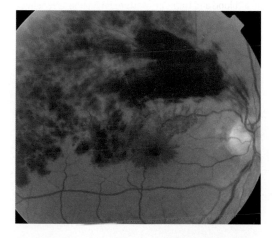

Fig. 27.21 Branch retinal vein occlusion (BRVO)—superficial flame-shaped hemorrhages and deeper intraretinal hemorrhages in the distribution of the occluded superotemporal retinal vein.

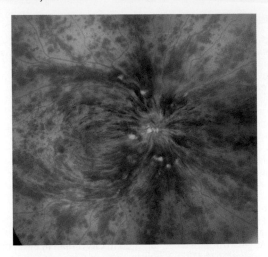

Fig. 27.22 Hemorrhagic central retinal vein occlusion (CRVO)—extensive flame-shaped and blot hemorrhages in a "blood and thunder" pattern indicating severe hemorrhagic CRVO. CWSs are suggestive of ischemia, and retinal folds represent edema. The optic disc is swollen and has multiple superficial hemorrhages.

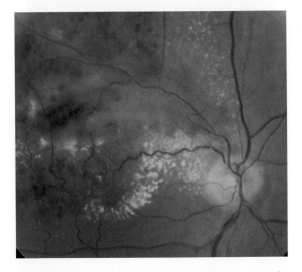

Fig. 27.23 Branch retinal vein occlusion (BRVO), 4 months after the initial presentation in Fig. 27.21. Most of the hemorrhages have resolved. Telangiectasis, residual hemorrhages, venous sheathing, and hard exudates, representing retinal edema and vascular incompetence, are present.

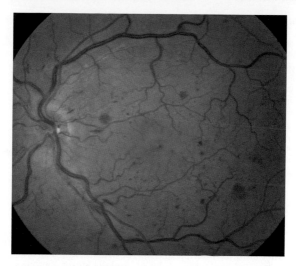

Fig. 27.24 Mild, nonhemorrhagic central retinal vein occlusion (CRVO). Flame-shaped and dot and blot hemorrhages, telangiectasis, and vascular tortuosity are present in all quadrants, suggestive of CRVO. The optic disc is hyperemic and has fine collateral vessels.

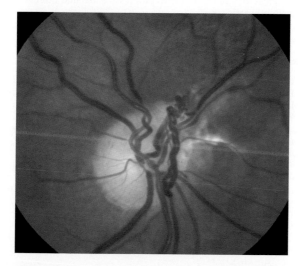

Fig. 27.25 Large optic disc collateral vessels are present in this patient with an old CRVO. In contrast to new vessels, collateral vessels do not leak or cause hemorrhage.

Risk Factors for Retinal Vein Occlusion

◆ Age
◆ Systemic hypertension
◆ Cardiovascular disease
◆ Obesity
◆ Hypercoagulable states
◆ Hyperviscosity syndromes
◆ Diabetes mellitus
◆ Sickle cell hemoglobinopathies—rare
◆ Glaucoma
◆ Retinal vasculitis

◆ Retinal Arterial Macroaneurysm

Retinal arterial macroaneurysms are acquired, abnormal saccular dilatations of retinal arteries. They are often multiple and may be bilateral in 10% of affected individuals. Retinal macroaneurysms often undergo spontaneous sclerosis and closure.

Symptoms

◆ Acute painless loss of vision due to vitreous or retinal hemorrhage
◆ Chronic painless loss of vision due to progressive macular edema
◆ May be asymptomatic

Fundus Features

◆ Red round vascular lesion, measuring 100 to 500 μm, on or adjacent to a retinal artery (**Fig. 27.26**). The lesions may be solitary or multiple, and unilateral or bilateral.
◆ Hemorrhage (**Fig. 27.27**)
    ◦ Retinal
    ◦ Subretinal
    ◦ Subhyaloid
    ◦ Intravitreal
◆ Retinal edema
◆ Hard exudates—often occur in a circinate pattern centered on the macroaneurysm
◆ Capillary telangiectasis
◆ Vascular sheathing
◆ Retinal vascular occlusion

Conditions Associated with Retinal Macroaneurysm

◆ Systemic hypertension—60%
◆ Retinal vasculopathies (e.g., Coats disease, Leber military aneurysms)
◆ Septic emboli
◆ Idiopathic

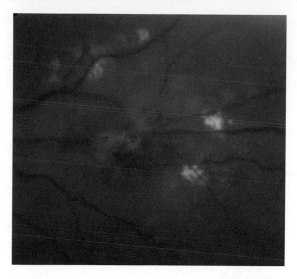

Fig. 27.26 Retinal macroaneurysms with surrounding retinal edema and hard exudates. Focal chorioretinal scars of prior retinal laser photocoagulation are present.

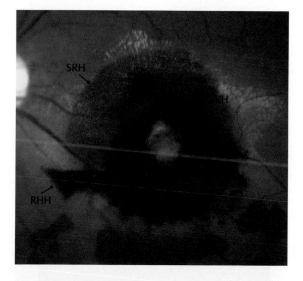

Fig. 27.27 Retinal macroaneurysm (MA) causing hemorrhages at various layers, including subretinal (SRH), retinal (RH), and retrohyaloid (RHH) hemorrhages. Presence of fine hard exudates indicates chronic leakage.

◆ Carotid Artery Disease (Ocular Ischemic Syndrome)

Retinal manifestations of carotid artery disease may be due to embolization to the retinal vasculature or to the ocular ischemic syndrome. Retinal arterial embolism is discussed earlier in this chapter. Ocular ischemic syndrome is usually associated with greater than 90% stenosis of the carotid artery.

Symptoms

◆ Gradual onset of visual loss
◆ Impaired dark adaptation
◆ Periocular and periorbital pain—pain improves on lying down

Fundus Features

◆ Flame-shaped and blot hemorrhages (**Fig. 27.28**)—Typically, retinal hemorrhages are prominent in the equatorial region.
◆ Microaneurysms
◆ Cotton-wool spots
◆ Narrowed retinal arteries
◆ Dilated (but often not tortuous) retinal veins. This contrasts with retinal vein occlusion where the veins are both dilated and tortuous.
◆ Retinal and optic disc neovascularization

Other Ophthalmic Features

◆ Ocular hypotony
◆ Anterior chamber flare
◆ Iris atrophy
◆ Iris neovascularization

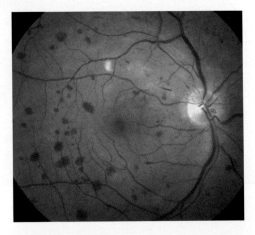

Fig. 27.28 Slow-flow retinopathy due to carotid artery stenosis. The retinal veins are dark and dilated (not tortuous). Multiple intraretinal blot, flame-shaped, and dot hemorrhages are present, along with CWSs.

◆ Hyperlipidemia

Hyperlipidemia is associated with general atheromatous disease and, therefore, with its sequelae in the retina. In addition, severe hyperlipidemia may result in slow retinal blood flow, causing vascular tortuosity, dilatation, and mild retinal hemorrhages. In severe hyperlipidemia, the retinal vessels appear salmon-pink or yellow rather than red (**Figs. 27.29 and 27.30**).

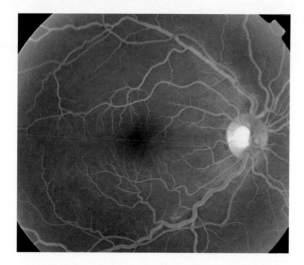

Fig. 27.29 Salmon-pink and tortuous retinal vessels in a 32-year-old African-American male with severe hypertriglyceridemia.

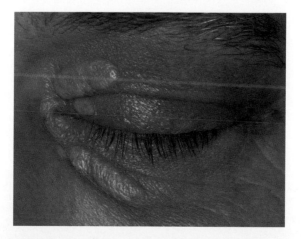

Fig. 27.30 Xanthelasma of the eyelid skin in a patient with hyperlipidemia.

Pearls

- Patients with grade IV hypertensive retinopathy are at significantly increased risk of cardiovascular and cerebrovascular morbidity and mortality. They require urgent management of their hypertension.

- In patients with diabetes, poorly controlled hypertension exacerbates diabetic retinopathy. Blood pressure control is an integral part of managing patients with diabetic retinopathy.

- Retinal vein occlusion primarily affects individuals of 50 years of age or older. Young patients with severe or bilateral retinal vein occlusion require further evaluation for possible underlying disease, including hypercoagulable states and systemic vasculitis.

◆ Human Immunodeficiency Virus (HIV)/Acquired Immunodeficiency Syndrome (AIDS)

Human Immunodeficiency Virus Retinopathy

HIV retinopathy is a form of microvascular retinopathy that is usually asymptomatic and self-limiting.

Fundus Features (Fig. 28.1)

◆ Cotton-wool spots
◆ Retinal hemorrhages
◆ Microaneurysms
◆ Retinal vasculitis

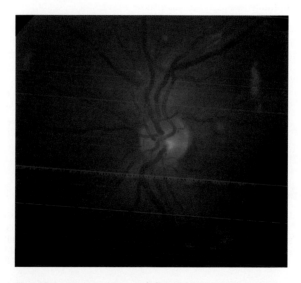

Fig. 28.1 Human immunodeficiency virus (HIV) retinopathy—multiple cotton-wool spots and minor hemorrhages in a patient with recently diagnosed HIV.

Ophthalmic Manifestations of AIDS

◆ Retina and choroid
  ◦ Cytomegalovirus (CMV) retinitis
  ◦ Herpes zoster (HZV) retinitis
  ◦ Herpes simplex (HSV) retinitis
  ◦ Progressive outer retina necrosis (PORN)—HSV, HZV
  ◦ Toxoplasma retinochoroiditis
  ◦ Syphilis chorioretinitis
  ◦ Candida chorioretinitis/endophthalmitis
  ◦ Pneumocystis chorioretinitis
  ◦ Cryptococcus chorioretinitis
◆ Neuro-ophthalmic
  ◦ Optic disc edema
    ◆ Papilledema—central nervous system (CNS) lymphoma, abscesses, and mass lesions
    ◆ Infiltration—lymphoma, infections
    ◆ Optic neuropathy
  ◦ Cranial nerve palsies
  ◦ Nystagmus
  ◦ Encephalopathy
  ◦ Visual field defects
◆ Orbit
  ◦ Lymphoma
  ◦ Kaposi sarcoma
◆ Uveitis—immune reconstitution uveitis
◆ Cornea and conjunctiva
  ◦ Microsporidium keratoconjunctivitis
  ◦ Kaposi sarcoma
  ◦ Squamous cell carcinoma
◆ Eyelids
  ◦ Herpes zoster
  ◦ Molluscum contagiosum
  ◦ Kaposi sarcoma

◆ Cytomegalovirus Infections

Cytomegalovirus Retinitis

CMV retinitis is the most common ocular opportunistic infection in patients with AIDS. CMV retinitis is a full-thickness retinal necrosis that typically occurs when the CD4 count is below 50/µL. It can also occur in HIV-negative individuals who are immunocompromised (e.g., posttransplant patients and patients with leukemia).

Symptoms

◆ Asymptomatic
◆ Floaters
◆ Painless loss of vision

Fundus Features

◆ Retinal necrosis—granular or patchy yellow-white opacified areas of variable size with irregular borders (**Fig. 28.2**)
◆ Retinal hemorrhages (**Fig. 28.3**)
◆ Exudates
◆ Vascular sheathing (**Fig. 28.4**)
◆ Mild, variable overlying vitritis
◆ Hyper/hypopigmented atrophic scars
◆ Diffuse/patchy retinal pigmentary changes—old, inactive scars of CMV retinitis
◆ Retinal breaks
◆ Retinal detachment

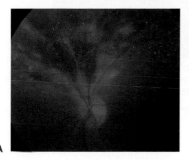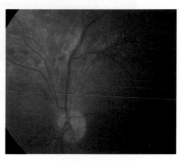

A   B

Fig. 28.2 Cytomegalovirus (CMV) retinitis. (**A**) Extensive hemorrhages, yellow-cream areas of active retinitis, and vascular sheathing in a patient with AIDS and CD4 count of 10/μL. (**B**) Regression of CMV retinitis 4 months after initiation of treatment for HIV and CMV. The retina is diffusely atrophic with underlying pigmentary changes.

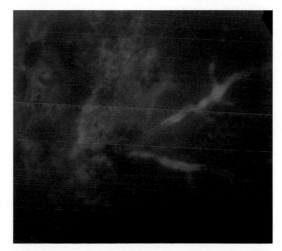

Fig. 28.3 Active CMV retinitis—extensive retinal hemorrhages, yellow-cream–colored granular and patchy areas of retinitis, and vascular sheathing.

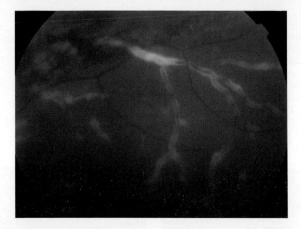

Fig. 28.4   Extensive vascular sheathing ("frosted branch" angiitis) and CMV retinitis in a patient with AIDS.

Differential Diagnosis

◆ Cotton-wool spots
◆ HZV or HSV retinitis
◆ Branch retinal vein occlusion
◆ Diabetic retinopathy
◆ Myelinated nerve fibers

Congenital Cytomegalovirus Infection

Congenital infection with CMV is the most common congenital infection in humans, occurring in 1% of newborns. Over 90% of cases remain asymptomatic. Transmission is usually transplacental.

Fundus Features

- ◆ Active
  - ○ Retinitis/choroiditis—less severe than acquired CMV retinitis
    - ◆ Flat, whitish retinal lesions, retinal hemorrhages
  - ○ Vitritis
  - ○ Optic neuritis
- ◆ Late
  - ○ Chorioretinal scars
  - ○ Pigmented retinopathy
  - ○ Optic atrophy
  - ○ Retinal detachment

Other Ophthalmic Features

- ◆ Microphthalmia
- ◆ Optic nerve hypoplasia
- ◆ Coloboma
- ◆ Cataract
- ◆ Glaucoma

◆ Herpes Zoster Virus (HZV) and Herpes Simplex Virus (HSV)

HZV and HSV Retinitis

HZV and HSV may cause retinitis characterized by white-creamy patches of retinal necrosis associated with vitritis (**Fig. 28.5**). A particularly severe form of retinitis

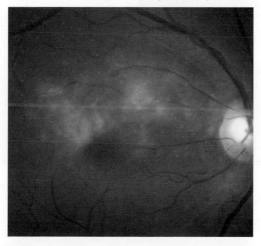

Fig. 28.5 Patchy, cream-colored areas of retinitis and segmental areas of arterial and venous sheathing in a patient with herpes retinitis.

is termed acute retinal necrosis (ARN). In early stages ARN may be asymptomatic. Without treatment, the prognosis is poor, and the fellow eye becomes involved in the majority of patients. A particularly severe form of HZV/HSV occurs in immunocompromised individuals and is termed progressive outer retinal necrosis (PORN).

Symptoms

◆ Asymptomatic in early stages
◆ Blurring/loss of vision
◆ Floaters
◆ Photophobia
◆ Ocular pain
◆ Eye redness

Fundus Features

◆ Retinitis—patchy peripheral areas of retinal whitening (necrosis) that become progressively confluent (**Fig. 28.6A**)
◆ Retinal vasculitis—sheathing of retinal vessels (**Fig. 28.6B**)
◆ Optic neuropathy (**Fig. 28.7**)
◆ Retinal hemorrhages
◆ Vitritis
◆ Anterior uveitis
◆ Late retinal detachment

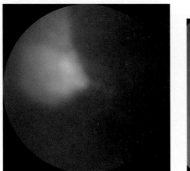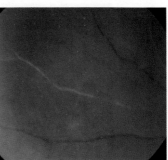

A   B

Fig. 28.6 Herpes zoster acute retinal necrosis (ARN). **(A)** Peripheral area of retinitis. **(B)** Peripheral retinal arteritis.

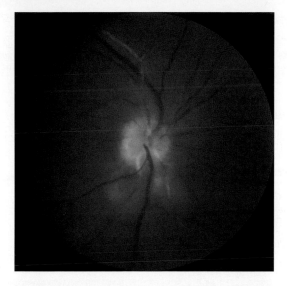

Fig. 28.7 Acute retinal necrosis (ARN)—optic neuropathy and retinal arteritis in a patient with ARN.

Congenital HZV and HSV Infection

Fundus Features

◆ Active
  ◦ Retinitis/choroiditis—less severe than ARN
  ◦ Vitritis
  ◦ Optic neuritis
◆ Late
  ◦ Chorioretinal scars
  ◦ Pigmented retinopathy
  ◦ Optic atrophy
  ◦ Vitreous opacity/mass

◆ Tuberculosis

Tuberculosis is caused by inhalation of airborne droplets containing *Mycobacterium tuberculosis*. The infection remains subclinical in over 90% of affected individuals.

Fundus Features

◆ Focal/multifocal chorioretinal lesions—small to medium-size (¼ to 1 disc diameter [DD]) yellow-white subretinal lesions (**Figs. 28.8 and 28.9**)
◆ Choroidal tuberculoma
◆ Retinal vasculitis
◆ Vitritis
◆ Optic disc swelling
  ◦ Optic papillitis
  ◦ Papilledema—TB lesions involving CNS
◆ Chronic uveitis
◆ Late chorioretinal scars

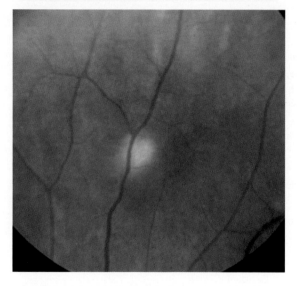

Fig. 28.8 Tuberculosis—focal yellow-cream–colored subretinal lesion representing choroidal infiltrate in a patient with tuberculosis.

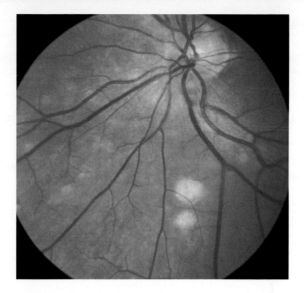

Fig. 28.9 Two yellowish focal choroidal infiltrates and multiple faint lesions of variable size in a patient with miliary tuberculosis.

Other Ophthalmic Features

- Eyelid lesions
- Chronic conjunctivitis
- Keratitis
- Scleritis/episcleritis
- Anterior uveitis—usually granulomatous
- Panuveitis
- Orbital tuberculoma

◆ Syphilis

Syphilis is a sexually transmitted disease caused by the spirochete *Treponema pallidum*. Fetal infection occurs following maternal spirochetemia.

Acquired Syphilis

Retinal and choroidal involvement is associated with secondary and tertiary syphilis.

Fundus Features

- ◆ Chorioretinitis (**Fig. 28.10**)
  - ◦ Characterized by areas of choroiditis with overlying retinal edema or necrosis, usually placoid or diffuse, but may be focal or multifocal
- ◆ Cotton-wool spots
- ◆ Flame-shaped hemorrhages/blot and dot hemorrhages
- ◆ Retinitis—focal or diffuse yellow-white areas associated with hemorrhage
- ◆ Retinal vasculitis—sheathing of retinal vessels, hemorrhages
- ◆ Retinal vascular occlusion, neovascularization
- ◆ Neuroretinitis
- ◆ Exudative retinal detachment
- ◆ Vitritis
- ◆ Choroidal neovascularization
- ◆ Optic disc swelling
  - ◦ Papillitis
  - ◦ Papilledema—CNS lesions
- ◆ Chronic uveitis
- ◆ Optic atrophy—Triad of bilateral optic atrophy, ptosis, and small irregular pupil is characteristic of tertiary syphilis.
- ◆ Late chorioretinal scars, pigmentary retinopathy, attenuated retinal vasculature (**Fig. 28.11**)

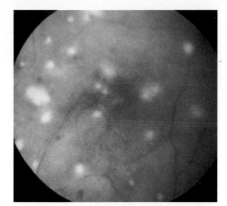

Fig. 28.10 Syphilitic posterior uveitis—multiple cream-colored choroidal lesions in a patient with secondary syphilis. The view is hazy due to vitritis.

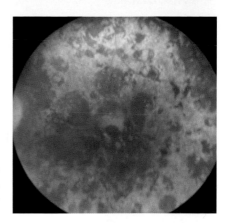

Fig. 28.11 Extensive patchy areas of pigmented chorioretinal scars in a patient with history of posterior uveitis and syphilis.

Other Ophthalmic Features

- ◆ Maculopapular lesions and nodules on eyelids
- ◆ Chronic conjunctivitis, conjunctival chancre
- ◆ Keratitis—interstitial; more common in congenital syphilis; often becomes symptomatic several years after birth
- ◆ Scleritis/episcleritis
- ◆ Iris nodules, roseate appearance, atrophy
- ◆ Dislocation of the lens
- ◆ Anterior uveitis
- ◆ Panuveitis
- ◆ Neuro-ophthalmic
  - ◦ Argyll Robertson pupil—small, irregular pupil that reacts poorly to light
  - ◦ Light-near dissociation—poor pupillary light reflex, preserved accommodative reflex
  - ◦ Cranial nerve palsies
  - ◦ Optic neuritis, papilledema, atrophy
  - ◦ Visual field defects
  - ◦ Nystagmus

Congenital Syphilis

- Early
  - Chorioretinitis
  - Keratoconjunctivitis
- Late
  - Chorioretinal scars
  - Salt-and-pepper retinopathy
  - Attenuated retinal vasculature
  - Optic atrophy
  - Uveitis
  - Interstitial keratitis (IK)—Hutchinson triad: IK, deafness, Hutchinson teeth (peg-shaped incisors)

◆ Lyme Disease

Lyme disease is caused by the tick-borne spirochete, *Borrelia burgdorferi.* Systemic features include constitutional symptoms, inflammatory arthropathy, cardiac and neurologic abnormalities, and a characteristic erythematous (bull's-eye) skin lesion at the site of the tick bite, erythema chronicum migrans.

Fundus Features

- Neuroretinitis (**Fig. 28.12**)
- Chorioretinitis (**Fig. 28.13**)
- Retinitis
- Retinal vasculitis
- Retinal vascular occlusion
- Exudative retinal detachment
- Vitritis
- Panuveitis
- Optic neuritis
- Optic atrophy

Other Ophthalmic Features

- Conjunctivitis
- Scleritis
- Keratitis
- Anterior uveitis
- Cranial nerve palsies, especially VII

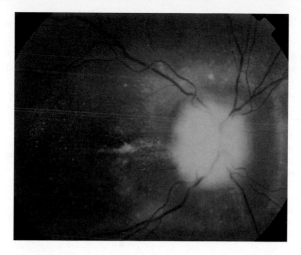

Fig. 28.12 Neuroretinitis in a patient with Lyme disease—optic disc swelling, peripapillary serous retinal detachment, and radial deposits of hard exudates are present.

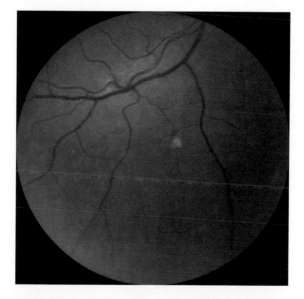

Fig. 28.13 Focal choroiditis in a patient with Lyme disease.

◆ Cat-Scratch Disease

Cat-scratch disease is a granulomatous infection caused by *Bartonella henselae*. It causes an acute or subacute neuroretinitis that is usually unilateral (90%).

Fundus Features

- Neuroretinitis (**Fig. 28.14**)
  - Optic disc swelling
  - Serous retinal detachment
  - Retinal edema
  - Macular star
- Chorioretinitis
- Focal retinitis
- Retinal vasculitis
- Retinal vascular occlusion
- Vitritis
- Optic neuritis
- Optic disc granuloma (**Fig. 28.15**)
- Optic atrophy—segmental or diffuse

Other Ophthalmic Features

- Conjunctivitis—Parinaud oculoglandular syndrome
- Scleritis
- Anterior uveitis
- Cranial nerve palsies

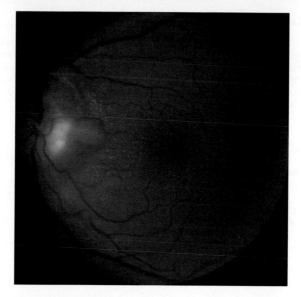

Fig. 28.14 Neuroretinitis associated with cat-scratch disease. The optic disc margin is blurred, and deposits of fine hard exudates are present in a radial pattern. Circumferential retinal folds (superior and temporal to the optic disc) suggest presence of peripapillary serous retinal detachment.

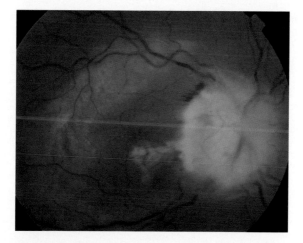

Fig. 28.15 Optic disc granuloma, retinal hemorrhages, and retinal edema in a patient with cat-scratch disease. The yellow-cream–colored patchy retinal lesion (temporal to the optic disc) represents an area of cloudy swelling caused by small retinal artery occlusion.

◆ Bacteremia

In patients with bacteremia, the retina may be affected by septic microemboliza-tion, deposition of immune complexes, disseminated intravascular coagulation, and bleeding abnormalities. Associated etiologies include bacterial endocarditis, indwelling catheterization, advanced malignancy, and severe infections of gastro-intestinal or urinary tract.

Symptoms

◆ Most often visually asymptomatic
◆ Blurred vision
◆ Floaters
◆ Ocular pain
◆ Photophobia
◆ Red eye

Fundus Features

◆ White-centered retinal hemorrhages—Roth spots
◆ Superficial flame-shaped and dot/blot retinal hemorrhages
◆ Cotton-wool spots
◆ Retinal/choroidal infiltrates (**Fig. 28.16**)
◆ Retinal/subretinal/choroidal abscess
◆ Focal or multifocal choroiditis
◆ Vitritis
◆ Endogenous endophthalmitis—clinically characterized by the development of hypopyon and vitritis (**Fig. 28.17**)

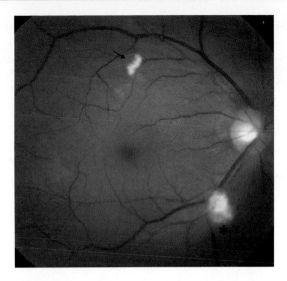

Fig. 28.16 Bacteremia—cotton-wool spot (*arrow*) and retinal infiltrate (*asterisk*) in a patient with subacute bacterial endocarditis.

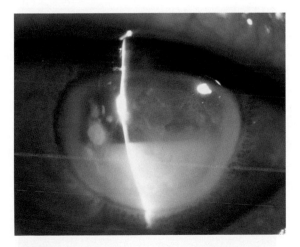

Fig. 28.17 Hypopyon in a patient with endogenous endophthalmitis, bacteremia, and history of intravenous drug abuse.

◆ Nocardiosis

Nocardiosis *(Nocardia asteroides)* occurs in immunosuppressed patients, and primarily affects the lungs and pleura. Hematogenous spread to the eye occurs in about 10% of cases (**Figs. 28.18 and 28.19**).

Fundus Features

◆ Retinal hemorrhage
◆ Retinal/subretinal abscess
◆ Choroidal abscess
◆ Chorioretinitis
◆ Vitritis

Other Ophthalmic Features

◆ Anterior uveitis
◆ Scleritis
◆ Keratitis
◆ Periorbital infection

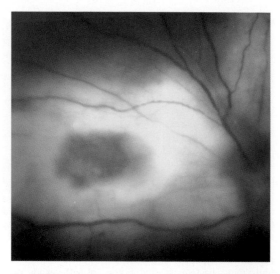

Fig. 28.18   Subretinal abscess in a patient with nocardiosis.

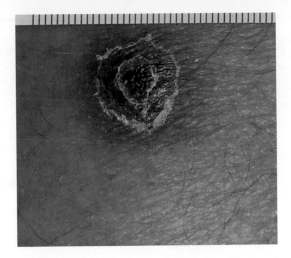

Fig. 28.19 Scaly, erythematous skin lesion with central area of necrosis in a patient with nocardiosis.

◆ Toxoplasmosis

Toxoplasmosis is an infection caused by the protozoan *Toxoplasma gondii*. The most common ocular presentation of toxoplasmosis is a unilateral retinochoroiditis characterized by a yellow-white focal area of retinitis often adjacent to an old chorioretinal scar, representing recurrence (**Fig. 28.20 and 28.21**). In most cases

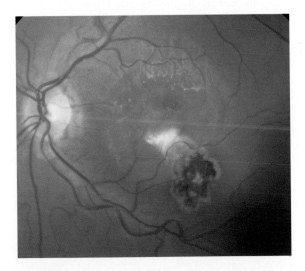

Fig. 28.20 Toxoplasma retinochoroiditis—focal whitish lesion with irregular borders, adjacent to an old pigmented chorioretinal scar.

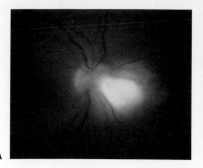
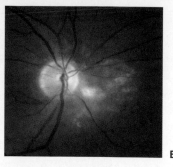

A   **B**

Fig. 28.21   Toxoplasma retinochoroiditis. **(A)** Active area of *Toxoplasma retinochoroiditis* adjacent to and involving the optic nerve head. The visual acuity was 20/60. **(B)** Peripapillary chorioretinal scar 3 months after treatment with systemic antibiotics and steroids. The visual acuity returned to 20/20.

the disease is a recurrence of congenital infection. In immunocompromised individuals the condition may be acquired, bilateral, and very severe. In AIDS patients, ocular toxoplasmosis is strongly associated with CNS toxoplasmosis.

Symptoms

◆ Blurring of vision
◆ Floaters
◆ Pain, photophobia, redness—if anterior uveitis is present
◆ Asymptomatic

Fundus Features

◆ Retinochoroiditis—often focal, white, fluffy lesion adjacent to old pigmented scar
◆ Focal retinal vasculitis (sheathing)
◆ Vascular occlusion
◆ Macular edema
◆ Serous retinal detachment
◆ Papillitis
◆ Vitritis—may obscure detailed view of the fundus; focal retinochoroiditis lesions may cause a "headlight in fog" appearance (**Fig. 28.22**)
◆ Panuveitis
◆ Old chorioretinal scar
◆ Necrotizing retinitis—in immunocompromised patient

Congenital Toxoplasmosis

◆ Chorioretinal scars—macula or periphery (**Fig. 28.23**)
◆ Vitreous opacities
◆ Cataract
◆ Microphthalmia
◆ Glaucoma

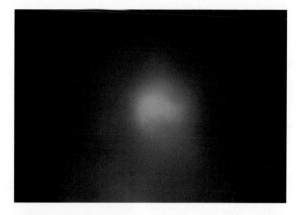

Fig. 28.22   Toxoplasma retinochoroiditis—"headlight in fog" appearance of focal area of retinochoroiditis, obscured by overlying vitreous haze due to vitritis.

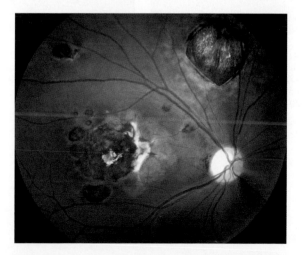

Fig. 28.23   Extensive pigmented chorioretinal scars involving the macula and the peripheral retina in a 26-year-old woman with history of congenital toxoplasmosis.

◆ Histoplasmosis

Histoplasmosis is caused by the fungus *Histoplasma capsulatum*. Acute systemic histoplasmosis is rarely associated with ocular involvement, such as granulomatous chorioretinitis and uveitis. More commonly, the retina is involved as part of the chronic ocular histoplasmosis syndrome (OHS). OHS occurs in otherwise asymptomatic individuals and is characterized by an absence of visible ocular inflammation or systemic abnormalities.

Fundus Features (Figs. 28.24, 28.25, and 28.26)

◆ "Histo spots"—multiple, focal, hyper- or hypopigmented chorioretinal scars measuring one third to one half of a DD.
◆ Peripapillary chorioretinal atrophy
◆ Peripheral linear or curvilinear streaks
◆ Choroidal neovascularization causing subretinal hemorrhage, especially in the macula

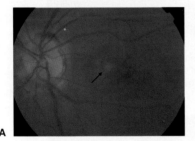 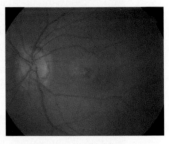

A   B

Fig. 28.24   Ocular histoplasmosis syndrome. **(A)** Peripapillary chorioretinal scarring and juxtafoveal choroidal neovascular membrane (CNV) (*arrow*) with small patch of subretinal hemorrhage in a 27-year-old woman. **(B)** Focal pigmented chorioretinal scar 6 months after laser photocoagulation of the CNV. The visual acuity improved from 20/70 to 20/25.

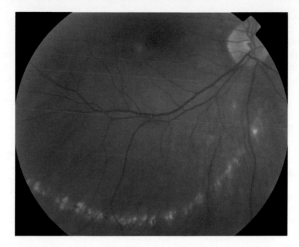

Fig. 28.25 Ocular histoplasmosis syndrome—multiple focal chorioretinal scars, in a curvilinear pattern, typically seen in ocular histoplasmosis syndrome.

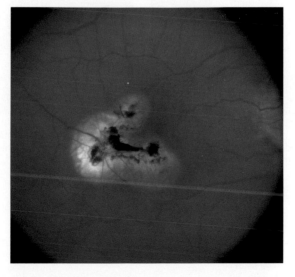

Fig. 28.26 Macular scar in a patient with ocular histoplasmosis syndrome and history of choroidal neovascularization.

◆ Cryptococcosis

Cryptococcus neoformans is a yeast that has a predilection for the CNS and is the most common cause of fungal meningitis. *C. neoformans* infection is more common in immunocompromised patients.

Fundus Features

- ◆ Multifocal choroiditis
  - ○ Discrete, variably sized, yellow-white lesions (**Fig. 28.27**)
  - ○ Predilection for the peripapillary region and optic disc (**Fig. 28.28**)
- ◆ Vitritis
- ◆ Retinal necrosis
- ◆ Vascular sheathing
- ◆ Exudative retinal detachment

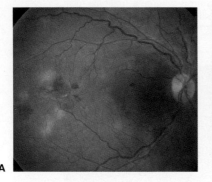 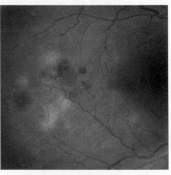

A   B

Fig. 28.27 Cryptococcosis. **(A)** Round, yellow-orange choroidal infiltrates of varying size and retinal hemorrhages in a patient with cryptococcus meningitis and AIDS. **(B)** Higher magnification photograph of the choroidal lesions.

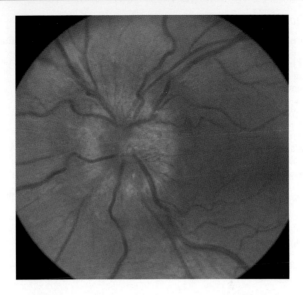

Fig. 28.28   Optic disc swelling in a patient with cryptococcus meningitis.

◆ Fungemia

In fungemia, infective microemboli become impacted within the choroidal and retinal circulations. The pathogens more commonly associated with fungemia include *Candida albicans* and other *Candida* species, *Aspergillus fumigatus, Blastomyces dermatitidis, Histoplasma capsulatum, Cryptococcus neoformans,* and *Coccidioides immitis.*

Symptoms

◆ Most often visually asymptomatic
◆ Blurred vision
◆ Floaters
◆ Ocular pain
◆ Photophobia
◆ Red eye

Fundus Features

◆ Chorioretinal infiltration—variably sized creamy-white lesions that may or may not be associated with vitritis (**Figs. 28.29 and 28.30**)
◆ Retinal hemorrhages
  ◦ Flame-shaped
  ◦ Dot and blot
  ◦ White-centered (pseudo-Roth spots)
◆ Cotton-wool spots
◆ Retinal vasculitis
◆ Retinal necrosis
◆ Retinal/subretinal/subhyaloid abscess
◆ Tractional retinal detachment
◆ Vitritis
◆ Vitreous opacities—"string of pearls"
◆ Endogenous endophthalmitis—severe vitritis, hypopyon (**Fig. 28.31**)

Other Ophthalmic Features

◆ Fungal corneal ulcer
◆ Anterior uveitis
◆ Scleritis

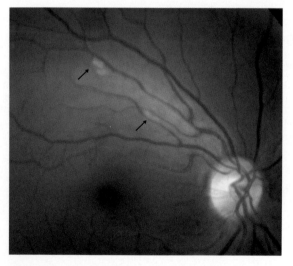

Fig. 28.29 Fungal infiltrates (*arrows*), resembling cotton-wool spots, in a patient with candida fungemia. The infiltrates resolved within 2 weeks of systemic antifungal therapy.

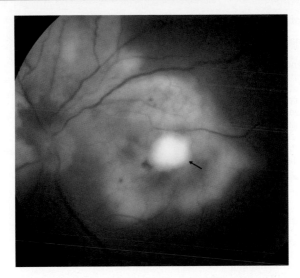

Fig. 28.30 Extensive subretinal aspergillus infiltrate in a patient with systemic aspergillosis, leukopenia, and chemotherapy for leukemia. Fungal infiltrate is seen breaking through the retina into the vitreous cavity (*arrow*).

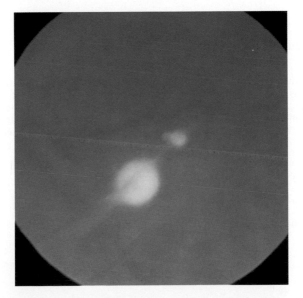

Fig. 28.31 Candida vitreous infiltrates ("fluff balls") and vitritis in a patient with endogenous endophthalmitis and systemic candidiasis.

Risk Factors for Fungal Chorioretinitis/Endophthalmitis

◆ Immunosuppressive therapy
◆ AIDS
◆ Intravenous hyperalimentation
◆ Intravenous drug abuse
◆ Chronic alcoholism
◆ Poorly controlled diabetes mellitus
◆ Prolonged antibiotic therapy
◆ Liver transplantation
◆ Advanced malignancy
◆ Major abdominal surgery
◆ Hemodialysis
◆ Prematurity

Differential Diagnosis of Fungal Chorioretinitis/Endophthalmitis

◆ Septic embolization due to bacteremia
◆ Disseminated intravascular coagulopathy (DIC)
◆ Bone marrow/fat/amniotic fluid embolization
◆ Viral retinitis
◆ Toxoplasma chorioretinitis
◆ Diabetic retinopathy
◆ Hypertensive retinopathy
◆ Sarcoidosis
◆ Cotton-wool spot—may mimic early fungal chorioretinal infiltration

◆ Toxocariasis

Ocular toxocariasis is caused by the larval nematode, *Toxocara canis.* It presents typically as a unilateral intraocular inflammation in a child or young adult. Systemic manifestations, such as visceral larval migrans, eosinophilia, and fever, are uncommon in ocular toxocariasis. Inflammation is worsened by the death of the nematode. Antihelminthic therapy is usually not effective in ocular disease.

Symptoms

◆ Painless loss of vision
◆ Floaters
◆ Photophobia

Fundus Features

- Chorioretinal granuloma—white, granulomatous mass in the macula or peripheral retina (**Figs. 28.32 and 28.33**)
- Vitritis
- Panuveitis
- Vitreoretinal bands
- Distortion of retinal vessels, macula, or optic disc (**Fig. 28.34**)
- Tractional retinal detachment
- Chorioretinal scar
- Leukokoria (white pupil)

Other Ophthalmic Features

- Secondary cataract
- Secondary glaucoma

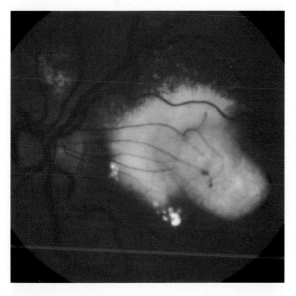

Fig. 28.32 Toxocara granuloma at the posterior pole.

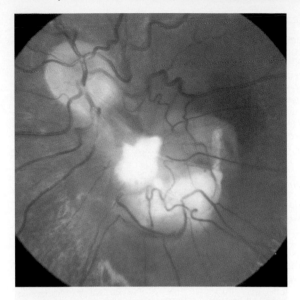

Fig. 28.33 Distortion of the retinal vessels, and preretinal and subretinal fibrosis in a patient with ocular toxocara.

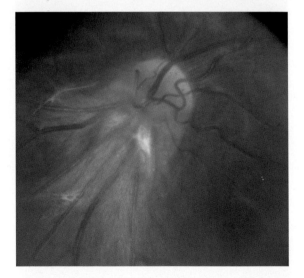

Fig. 28.34 Dragging of the optic disc and retinal vessels in a patient with peripheral toxocara granuloma.

◆ Cysticercosis

Cysticercosis is caused by *Cysticercus cellulosae,* the larval form of *Taenia solium.* Ocular involvement occurs in 20 to 40% of patients with systemic cysticercosis. It may be asymptomatic or cause blurring of vision, pain, photophobia and redness.

Fundus Features

- ◆ Subretinal or intravitreal *Cysticercus* cyst (**Fig. 28.35**)
- ◆ Chronic vitritis
- ◆ Retinal edema, hard exudates, hemorrhages
- ◆ Retinal vasculitis
- ◆ Chorioretinal scar
- ◆ Optic neuritis
- ◆ Papilledema—intracranial cysticercosis
- ◆ Optic atrophy

Other Ophthalmic Features

- ◆ *Cysticercus* cyst in anterior chamber
- ◆ Anterior uveitis
- ◆ Neuro-ophthalmologic
  - ○ Visual field defects—due to CNS lesion or optic neuropathy
  - ○ Cranial nerve palsies
- ◆ Orbital and lacrimal gland infiltration

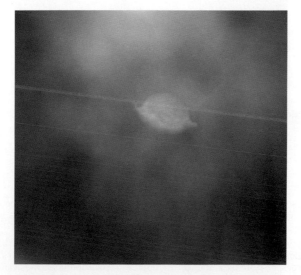

Fig. 28.35   Cysticercus cyst floating within the vitreous cavity.

◆ Pneumocystis Carinii

Systemic infection with *Pneumocystis carinii* may result in unilateral or bilateral choroidopathy characterized by the presence of multiple, variably sized, oval, pale cream-orange choroidal lesions, without vitreous inflammation (**Fig. 28.36**). Pneumocystis choroidopathy is usually asymptomatic. It occurs in patients with AIDS when the CD4 count falls below 200/µL. The condition was more common when use of prophylactic aerosolized pentamidine was widespread. Introduction of oral sulfamethoxazole/trimethoprim (SMZ-TMP) for the prophylaxis of *Pneumocystis* pneumonia has significantly reduced the occurrence of this choroidopathy.

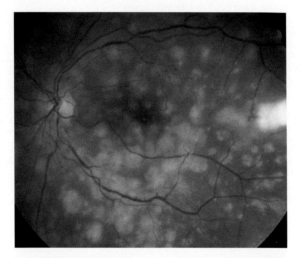

Fig. 28.36 Pneumocystis choroiditis—white-gray placoid choroidal infiltrates of variable size in a patient with *Pneumocystis* pneumonia and AIDS.

Pearls

- Regular retinal evaluation is indicated in patients with AIDS. Risk of CMV retinitis is highest when CD4 count is below 50/µL.

- Treatment of syphilitic chorioretinitis is similar to that of neurosyphilis and includes prolonged intravenous antibiotic therapy.

- Ocular involvement occurs in 20 to 30% of patients with fungemia if they are not receiving antifungal therapy. Occurrence of ocular involvement drops to about 3% in patients who are receiving treatment.

- In patients with fungemia, initial retinal examination is recommended to screen for early fungal chorioretinitis/endophthalmitis, as this may progress to loss of vision despite systemic antifungal therapy. Intraocular antifungal medications and surgery may become necessary if endophthalmitis develops.

29 Neurologic Disorders

◆ Papilledema

Papilledema refers to edema of the optic nerve head, secondary to the elevation of intracranial pressure. *Optic disc swelling* and *optic disc edema* describe swelling of the optic nerve in association with other conditions, such as optic neuritis, central retinal vein occlusion, anterior optic neuropathy, and severe hypertension. Papilledema is typically bilateral. Unilateral papilledema may occur in association with posterior subfrontal tumors (Foster-Kennedy syndrome) or when there has been preexisting optic atrophy or anomaly in one eye.

Symptoms

- ◆ Visually asymptomatic in most instances
- ◆ Transient visual obscurations, particularly on coughing, straining, and eye movement
- ◆ Severe chronic papilledema may result in optic atrophy with scotomas and loss of vision

Fundus Features (Figs. 29.1, 29.2, 29.3, and 29.4)

- ◆ Loss of spontaneous venous pulsation—an early sign that implies an intracranial pressure of >25 cm H_2O. Venous pulsation is absent in 20% of normal individuals.
- ◆ Hyperemia of the optic disc
- ◆ Blurring of the disc margin
- ◆ Elevation of the optic disc
- ◆ Optic disc and retinal hemorrhages
- ◆ Hard exudates
- ◆ Engorged retinal veins
- ◆ Peripapillary telangiectasis
- ◆ Retinal edema
- ◆ Chorioretinal folds
  - ◦ Peripapillary, circumferential folds (Paton folds)
  - ◦ Linear, curvilinear folds that extend over the macular region
- ◆ Peripapillary serous retinal detachment
- ◆ Optic disc leakage on fluorescein angiography

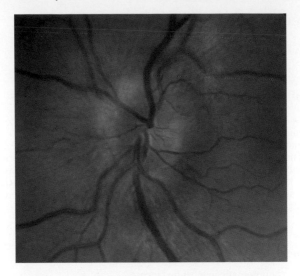

Fig. 29.1   Early-stage papilledema. The optic disc appears hyperemic. Margins are blurred, and fine telangiectasis is present.

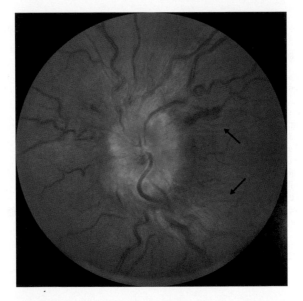

Fig. 29.2   Papilledema. The optic disc margins are blurred. The disc is hyperemic and elevated relative to the surrounding retina. Telangiectasis, vascular tortuosity, and hemorrhages are present. Chorioretinal folds (Paton folds) are seen temporal to the optic disc (*arrows*).

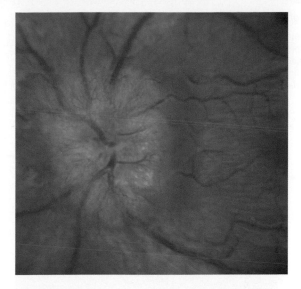

Fig. 29.3 Fully established papilledema. The optic disc is elevated and has extensive telangiectasis. Chorioretinal folds (Paton folds) are present.

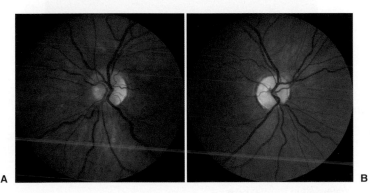

A   B

Fig. 29.4 Foster-Kennedy syndrome. **(A)** Mild papilledema with blurring of the nasal margin in the left eye of a patient with a right subfrontal meningioma. **(B)** Optic atrophy with temporal pallor of the right optic disc.

Features of Chronic Papilledema (Fig. 29.5)

◆ Prepapillary gliosis
◆ Gray appearance to the optic disc
◆ Telangiectasis
◆ Optic disc pallor (atrophy)
◆ Choroidal neovascularization and subretinal hemorrhage—rare association

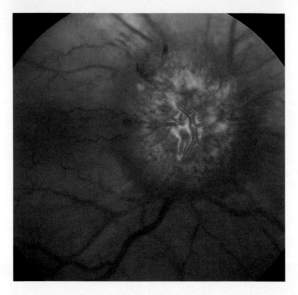

Fig. 29.5   Chronic papilledema. The optic disc is elevated and appears grayish due to early gliosis. Extensive telangiectasis is present.

Conditions Associated with Papilledema

◆ Space-occupying lesion of the central nervous system (CNS)
  ◦ Tumor
  ◦ Abscess
  ◦ Intracranial hemorrhage
◆ Decreased cerebrospinal fluid (CSF) reabsorption
  ◦ Venous sinus thrombosis
  ◦ Meningitis
  ◦ Subarachnoid hemorrhage
◆ Increased CSF production
  ◦ Choroidal plexus tumors
◆ Obstruction of the ventricular system
◆ Cerebral edema
  ◦ Ischemia
  ◦ Encephalitis
  ◦ Trauma
  ◦ Other
◆ Idiopathic intracranial hypertension (pseudotumor cerebri)

Differential Diagnosis

◆ Optic neuritis (papillitis)
◆ Central retinal vein occlusion
◆ Anterior ischemic optic neuropathy
◆ Toxic optic neuropathy
◆ Hereditary optic neuropathy
◆ Neuroretinitis (**Fig. 29.6**)
◆ Diabetic papillopathy
◆ Systemic hypertension
◆ Respiratory failure
◆ Carotid-cavernous fistula
◆ Optic disc/nerve infiltration
  ◦ Sarcoidosis
  ◦ Granuloma
  ◦ Lymphoma
  ◦ Leukemia
◆ Optic nerve or orbital tumors—optic nerve glioma, meningioma, lymphoma
◆ Ocular conditions
  ◦ Optic disc drusen (**Fig. 29.7**)
  ◦ Ocular hypotony
  ◦ Uveitis
  ◦ High hypermetropia

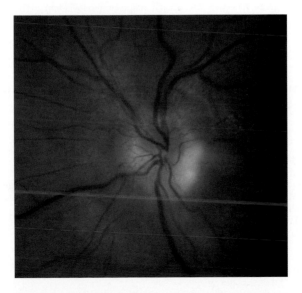

Fig. 29.6   Optic disc swelling in a patient with neuroretinitis and cat-scratch disease. The optic disc is hyperemic, and the margins are blurred due to peripapillary serous retinal detachment. Linear deposits of hard exudates are present.

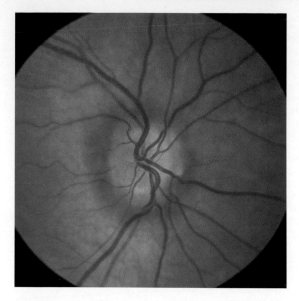

Fig. 29.7   Optic disc drusen mimicking papilledema. The optic disc is mildly elevated and has irregular "scalloped" margins, particularly nasally. Small, refractile hyaline deposits are visible at the nasal aspect of the disc. Vascular tortuosity, hemorrhages, and retinal edema are absent.

◆ Idiopathic Intracranial Hypertension (Pseudotumor Cerebri)

Idiopathic intracranial hypertension is characterized by:

◆ Papilledema (**Fig. 29.8**)
◆ Elevated intracranial pressure (>25 cm H_2O)
◆ Typically normal computed tomography (CT) scan and magnetic resonance imaging (MRI)
  ◦ Ventricles may appear small, however
◆ Normal cerebrospinal fluid composition

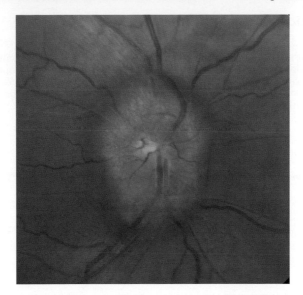

Fig. 29.8 Chronic papilledema in idiopathic intracranial hypertension. The optic disc is elevated and has a grayish tinge. Telangiectatic vessels are present on the surface of the disc.

The condition typically occurs in young, overweight females and most often presents with chronic headache (90%) that is exacerbated by straining, bending, and coughing. Some patients experience pulsatile tinnitus.

Fundus Features

◆ Bilateral papilledema, indistinguishable from papilledema caused by other diseases
◆ Long-standing cases develop features of chronic papilledema and optic atrophy.

Other Ophthalmic Features

◆ Diplopia
◆ Transient visual obscurations
◆ Cranial nerve VI palsy
◆ Visual field defects

◆ Optic Neuritis

Optic neuritis is characterized by acute, unilateral (or bilaterally asymmetrical) loss of vision due to demyelinating or inflammatory conditions of the optic nerve. The optic disc is swollen in 35% of cases (anterior optic neuritis). In 65% of cases, only the posterior part of the optic nerve is affected, and the optic disc appears normal initially.

Fundus Features

◆ Optic disc edema (**Fig. 29.9**)
◆ Hyperemic optic disc
◆ Telangiectasis over the disc
◆ Peripapillary hemorrhages
◆ Peripapillary retinal edema
◆ Perivenous sheathing—associated with multiple sclerosis
◆ Optic disc pallor—a late feature, developing about 6 weeks after the acute episode; represents atrophy that may be diffuse or segmental

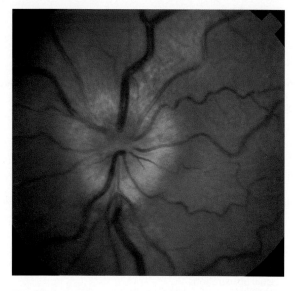

Fig. 29.9 Anterior optic neuritis. The disc is hyperemic, slightly elevated, and has blurred margins. The appearance is similar to papilledema, except that optic neuritis is associated with fewer hemorrhages and less vascular tortuosity. Optic neuritis is usually unilateral or asymmetrically bilateral. Unlike papilledema, the vision is often diminished, and scotomas, color vision abnormalities, and relative afferent pupillary defect are present in optic neuritis.

Other Ophthalmic Features

◆ Acute loss of vision
◆ Pain on eye movement
◆ Central, paracentral scotoma
◆ Color vision abnormalities
◆ Relative afferent pupillary defect

Conditions Associated with Optic Neuritis

◆ Demyelinating
  ◦ Idiopathic
  ◦ Multiple sclerosis
  ◦ Neuromyelitis optica (Devic's disease)
  ◦ Acute disseminated encephalopathy
◆ Inflammatory
  ◦ Autoimmune
    ◆ Systemic lupus erythematosus and other collagen vascular diseases
  ◦ Sarcoidosis
  ◦ Infections
    ◆ Syphilis
    ◆ Lyme disease
    ◆ Tuberculosis
    ◆ Viral—Herpes zoster, measles, mumps, Epstein-Barr
  ◦ Postvaccination
  ◦ Orbital cellulitis

◆ Ischemic Optic Neuropathy

Ischemic optic neuropathy (ION) may be anterior (optic disc swelling) or posterior (no optic disc swelling), arteritic (25%) or nonarteritic (75%). ION usually affects individuals over 55 years of age and typically presents as unilateral painless loss of vision. The contralateral side may become affected within weeks to months.

Fundus Features

◆ "Pale" swelling of the optic disc—as opposed to "pink" swelling of papilledema and optic neuritis (**Fig. 29.10**)
◆ Cotton-wool spots
◆ Splinter hemorrhages on the optic disc
◆ Attenuated blood vessels
◆ Features of chronic hypertensive retinopathy or retinal vasculitis may be present.

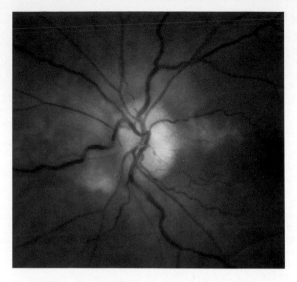

Fig. 29.10 Anterior ischemic optic neuropathy (AION). Pale swelling of the optic disc, characteristic of AION, is present. Patchy areas of gray-white cloudy edema, indicating acute ischemia, can be seen in the adjacent retina.

Other Ophthalmic Features

◆ Acute, initially unilateral, painless loss of vision
◆ Altitudinal visual field defects—characteristic of anterior ischemic optic neuropathy
◆ Abnormal color vision
◆ Relative afferent pupillary defect
◆ Optic atrophy—late feature

Systemic Conditions Predisposing to Ischemic Optic Neuropathy

◆ Nonarteritic ION
  ◦ Hypertension
  ◦ Acute hypotension
  ◦ Diabetes
  ◦ Malignancy
  ◦ Hyperviscosity syndromes
  ◦ Hypercoagulable states
  ◦ Hemoglobinopathies (rare)
  ◦ Migraine
◆ Arteritic ION
  ◦ Giant cell arteritis
  ◦ Systemic lupus erythematosus
  ◦ Polyarteritis nodosa
  ◦ Syphilis
  ◦ Radiation

◆ Toxic/Nutritional Optic Neuropathy

Optic neuropathy resulting from nutritional deficiency or toxic exposure is usually associated with bilateral, progressive, painless loss of vision with central or cecocentral scotoma.

Fundus Features (Fig. 29.11)

- ◆ Mild to moderate disc edema—usually in acute anterior cases
- ◆ Splinter hemorrhages at the optic disc
- ◆ Optic atrophy—late feature

Other Ophthalmic Features

- ◆ Bilateral, symmetrical, painless loss of vision
- ◆ Central/cecocentral scotoma
- ◆ Abnormal color vision
- ◆ Relative afferent pupillary defect—in cases with asymmetric involvement of the optic nerves

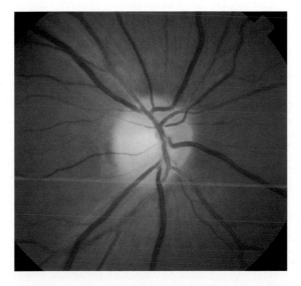

Fig. 29.11   Toxic optic neuropathy in a patient with methanol toxicity. The optic disc appears somewhat featureless, with diminished number of capillaries on the disc surface. Temporal pallor and mild blurring of margins are present.

Drugs/Chemicals Associated with Toxic Optic Neuropathy

- ◆ Drugs
  - ○ Ethambutol, isoniazid, amiodarone, chloramphenicol, sulfonamides, cisplatin, vincristine, penicillamine, hydroxyquinolines, barbiturates
- ◆ Methanol
- ◆ Ethylene glycol
- ◆ Heavy metals
  - ○ Lead
  - ○ Thallium
  - ○ Mercury
- ◆ Organophosphates
- ◆ Aniline dyes
- ◆ Nutritional deficiency (tobacco-alcohol amblyopia)
  - ○ B_{12}, folate, thiamine
  - ○ Tobacco—cigar and pipe

◆ Hereditary Optic Neuropathy

Leber Hereditary Optic Neuropathy (LHON)

Leber hereditary optic neuropathy (LHON) typically affects males 10 to 30 years of age. Women account for 10% of cases. LHON is associated with several mitochondrial DNA mutations, most frequently at the 11778 position. The condition is transmitted by mitochondrial DNA inherited from the mother.

Fundus Features (Fig. 29.12)

- ◆ Hyperemic, elevated optic disc (pseudo-edema)—Optic disc may appear normal in early stages.
- ◆ Peripapillary telangiectasis
- ◆ Thickening of peripapillary retina
- ◆ Tortuosity of medium-sized retinal arterioles
- ◆ Absence of leakage on fluorescein angiography
- ◆ Optic atrophy—late feature

Other Ophthalmic Features

- ◆ Acute painless loss of vision—initially unilateral, later bilateral
- ◆ Central, cecocentral scotoma
- ◆ Abnormal color vision
- ◆ Relative afferent pupillary defect—in cases with asymmetric involvement of the optic nerves
- ◆ Variable final visual acuity—usually 20/80 to 20/200

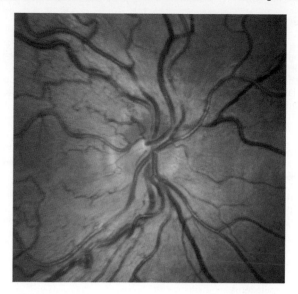

Fig. 29.12   Leber hereditary optic neuropathy (LHON). The optic disc is hyperemic with mild blurring of the margins. Peripapillary telangiectasis, and tortuosity of the larger vessels are present.

Dominant Optic Atrophy

Fundus Features

◆ Bilateral segmental disc pallor—wedge-shaped excavation

Other Ophthalmic Features

◆ Mild to moderate bilateral visual loss
◆ Central, cecocentral scotoma; binasal or bitemporal visual field defects
◆ Abnormal color vision (blue—yellow dyschromatopsia)
◆ Inverted color visual fields (blue field falls within the red field)
◆ Paradoxical pupillary reaction—pupillary constriction in dim light
◆ Nystagmus

Autosomal Recessive Optic Atrophy

Autosomal recessive optic atrophy usually occurs in association with other systemic abnormalities, such as pyramidal tract signs, ataxia, and mental retardation.

◆ Optic Nerve Atrophy (Fig. 29.13)

Optic atrophy represents damage to the retinal ganglion cells and their axons. It may result from damage to any portion of the cells, from cell bodies within the retina to their axon terminals at the lateral geniculate body. Optic atrophy is usually associated with loss of visual acuity, scotoma, abnormal color vision, and afferent pupillary defect.

Fundus Features

◆ Optic disc pallor—may be diffuse or segmental
◆ Loss of capillaries in the optic disc
◆ Attenuated vessels
◆ Loss of optic disc "substance"
◆ Sharp, clear margins (except when secondary to chronic papilledema)

Conditions Associated with Optic Nerve Atrophy

◆ Chronic papilledema
◆ Ischemic optic neuropathy
◆ Optic neuritis—demyelinating, inflammatory, infectious
◆ Toxic/nutritional optic neuropathy
◆ Hereditary optic neuropathy
◆ Optic nerve trauma
◆ Optic nerve compression
◆ Radiation optic neuropathy
◆ Optic chiasm compression, tumors, vascular occlusion, radiation, trauma
◆ Optic tract compression, tumors, vascular occlusion, radiation, trauma
◆ Meningitis
◆ Ocular
  ○ Severe acute or chronic glaucoma
  ○ Severe retinal disease

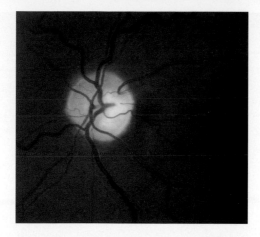

Fig. 29.13 Optic atrophy. The optic disc appears pale, and the margins are sharp and clear. There is loss of surface capillaries.

◆ Optic Disc Anomalies

Optic Disc Drusen (Fig. 29.14)

Optic disc drusen are yellow, refractile, often calcified nodules located within the optic nerve head. They may be superficial and hence visible, or deeply buried and not directly visible. Optic disc drusen are present in 1% of the general population and are usually asymptomatic. They may be sporadic, or have autosomal dominant inheritance. Optic disc drusen are more prevalent in the white race and are bilateral in 75% of cases. Differential diagnosis of optic disc drusen includes causes of optic disc swelling, such as papilledema.

Fundus Features

- ◆ Optic disc
  - ○ Elevated disc, often small
  - ○ Irregular margin
  - ○ Superficial drusen are visible as refractile nodules—Buried drusen are not directly visible.
  - ○ Anomalous vascular branching (e.g., trifurcation of central retinal vasculature and vascular loops)
  - ○ Optic disc or retinal hemorrhage may rarely be present.
  - ○ Absence of disc surface hyperemia or telangiectasia
  - ○ Absence of leakage on fundus fluorescein angiogram
  - ○ Autofluorescence on red-free viewing
  - ○ High echogenicity on B-scan ultrasound due to calcification
  - ○ Calcified optic nerve head lesion on CT scan
  - ○ Ischemic optic neuropathy
  - ○ Optic atrophy
- ◆ Subretinal neovascularization
- ◆ Angioid streaks (**Fig. 29.15**)
- ◆ Pigment retinopathy (e.g., retinitis pigmentosa)

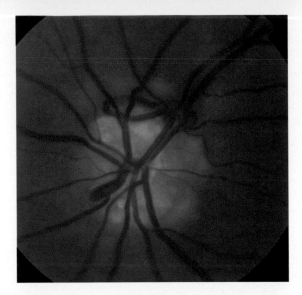

Fig. 29.14 Optic disc drusen. The optic disc is mildly elevated and has irregular "scalloped" margins. Small, refractile hyaline deposits are visible. The optic disc cup is absent, and there is anomalous branching of the blood vessels. Vascular tortuosity, hemorrhages, and retinal edema are absent.

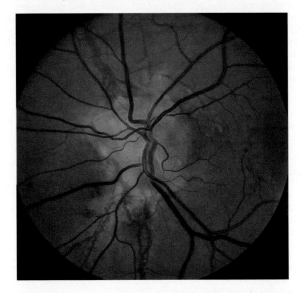

Fig. 29.15 Optic disc drusen may occasionally be associated with angioid streaks. Dark red, irregular subretinal bands (angioid streaks) are present around the optic disc and radiate toward the periphery. The optic disc is elevated, has hyaloid deposits, and irregular "scalloped" margins (optic disc drusen).

Other Ophthalmic Features

◆ Usually asymptomatic
◆ Transient visual obscurations
◆ Mild visual loss
◆ Enlarged blind spot and scotomas
◆ Relative afferent pupillary defect

Temporal Crescent (Fig. 29.16)

Temporal crescent is a commonly occurring, benign condition characterized by a small crescentic area of chorioretinal hypoplasia affecting the temporal side of the optic nerve head. It is visually inconsequential and is often associated with myopia.

Differential Diagnosis

◆ Pathologic myopia
◆ Ocular histoplasmosis syndrome
◆ Trauma
◆ Angioid streak
◆ Peripapillary choroidal neovascularization

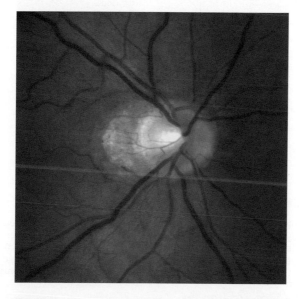

Fig. 29.16   A temporal peripapillary crescent of chorioretinal atrophy (shown here in the right eye) is a frequent finding and has no visual significance. It occurs more commonly in myopic individuals.

Tilted Optic Disc (Fig. 29.17)

Tilted optic disc is present in 2% of the general population and is usually bilateral. It represents an oblique entrance of the optic nerve into the eye. Tilted optic discs are visually asymptomatic but may be associated with the following:

◆ Astigmatism
◆ Myopia
◆ Abnormal retinal vascular pattern
◆ Hypopigmentation of the fundus—typically inferonasal or inferior fundus
◆ Upper temporal field defects that do not respect the midline

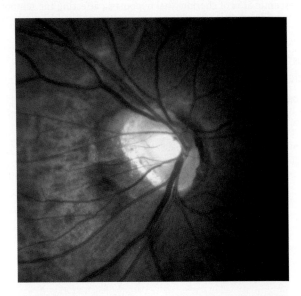

Fig. 29.17   Tilted optic disc in a right eye. The optic disc appears oval, because the nerve enters the globe obliquely. The blood vessels are nasally displaced compared with a normal disc. Peripapillary atrophy is a frequent finding.

High Hypermetropia

In highly hypermetropic eyes the optic disc appears small and crowded. The disc margin may appear slightly elevated due to overcrowding by nerve fibers entering the nerve, but it remains sharp. The optic disc cup is small or absent. In a hypermetropic optic disc, unlike papilledema, there are no retinal hemorrhages or gross vascular tortuosity, and the venous pulse is present in the majority of cases.

Myopic Optic Disc (Fig. 29.18)

In low and moderate myopia the appearance of the optic disc is normal. In high (pathologic) myopia the optic disc appears large, is often tilted, and has a shallow, enlarged cup. Peripapillary chorioretinal atrophy and straightening of temporal vessels are characteristic features.

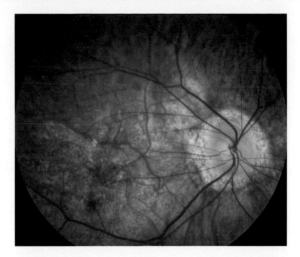

Fig. 29.18 Myopic optic disc in a right eye—large optic disc, peripapillary atrophy, straightening of the temporal blood vessels, and diffuse chorioretinal atrophy with visible choroidal vessels in a patient with high myopia.

Optic Disc Hypoplasia (Fig. 29.19)

Optic disc hypoplasia is characterized by a small anomalous optic disc that is often tilted. The condition is bilateral in 80% of cases. Optic disc hypoplasia may be segmental or complete. It may be associated with midline or hemispheric brain defects, hypothalamic dysfunction, and basal encephalocele.

Fundus Features

◆ Small optic disc—⅓ to ½ the normal size
◆ Segmental or complete hypoplasia
◆ Normal-size blood vessels that appear large relative to the disc
◆ Variable degree of tilting of the optic disc
◆ Yellow peripapillary halo surrounded by ring of hyper/hypopigmentation (double ring sign)

Other Ophthalmic Features

◆ Reduced vision—ranging from near-normal vision to severe visual loss
◆ Amblyopia
◆ Visual field defects—peripheral, arcuate, cecocentral scotomas
◆ Nystagmus—usually pendular

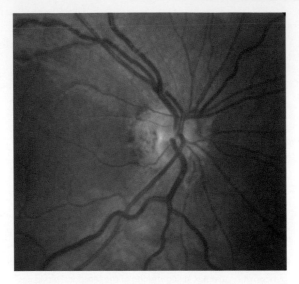

Fig. 29.19   Optic nerve hypoplasia. The optic disc is small, measuring approximately 750 μm (six times the caliber of the retinal vein). Characteristic peripapillary ring of atrophy and pigmentation is present.

Conditions Associated with Optic Disc Hypoplasia

◆ Septo-optic dysplasia (de Morsier syndrome)—especially if disc hypoplasia is bilateral
◆ Maternal diabetes mellitus
◆ Maternal drugs—antiepileptic medications, quinine, lysergic acid diethylamide (LSD)
◆ Maternal alcohol abuse
◆ Congenital tumor—optic glioma, craniopharyngioma

Optic Disc Coloboma (Fig. 29.20)

Optic disc coloboma is a deep excavation of the optic disc, often resulting from incomplete closure of the embryonic fissure (**Fig. 29.1**). In 90% of affected individuals, the condition is unilateral. The mode of inheritance is autosomal recessive in most cases. Bilateral cases may have autosomal dominant inheritance.

Fundus Features

◆ Deep excavation of optic disc
◆ Coloboma of inferonasal retina, choroid, iris, lens, and zonule (**Fig. 29.22**)
◆ Retinal detachment
◆ Remnants of fetal hyaloid system—persistent fetal vasculature

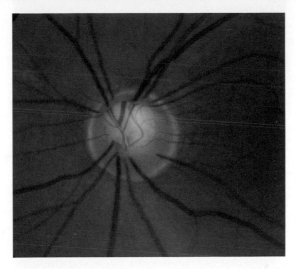

Fig. 29.20 Optic disc coloboma. Deep excavation of the optic disc is present.

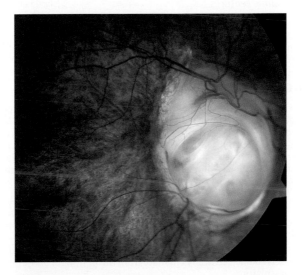

Fig. 29.21 Large optic disc coloboma—extensive excavation of the optic disc with distortion of the remaining optic disc tissue. Optic disc coloboma is a developmental, nonprogressive abnormality of the optic disc that is associated with variable degree of visual loss.

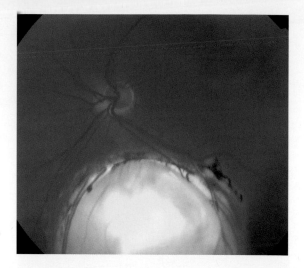

Fig. 29.22 Large chorioretinal coloboma, representing incomplete closure of the embryonic fissure, characteristically involving the inferior fundus.

Other Ophthalmic Features

◆ Poor vision
◆ Visual field defects
◆ Nystagmus
◆ Relative afferent pupillary defect—varying degree

Morning Glory Optic Disc

"Morning glory" optic disc anomaly is a typically unilateral funnel-shaped excavation or elevation of the optic disc and peripapillary chorioretinal layers (**Fig. 29.23**). "Morning glory" optic disc may be associated with basal encephalocele and renal disease. Renal disease is more typical of the papillorenal syndrome, in which the optic disc is atrophic and excavated, and may resemble the morning glory anomaly (**Fig. 29.24**). In papillorenal syndrome optic disc abnormalities are usually bilateral, but may be asymmetric.

Fundus Features

◆ Optic disc—enlarged, orange-gray color, may be elevated or recessed
◆ Blood vessels characteristically emanate from the periphery of the disc ("wheel-spokes" vasculature)
◆ Peripapillary area of staphyloma
◆ Chorioretinal pigmentation surrounding the disc
◆ Prepapillary glial tissue
◆ Secondary retinal conditions
  ◦ Serous retinal detachment
  ◦ Rhegmatogenous retinal detachment
  ◦ Choroidal neovascularization

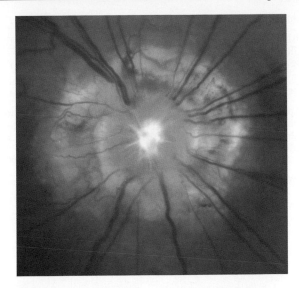

Fig. 29.23 "Morning glory" optic disc—enlarged, salmon-gray color, elevated optic disc with irregular margins. Prepapillary glial tissue and peripapillary chorioretinal atrophy and pigmentation are present. The blood vessels emanate from the periphery of the disc in a "wheel-spokes" pattern.

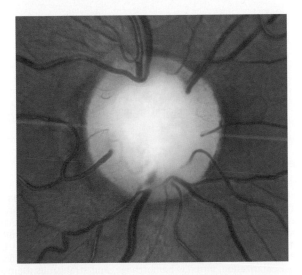

Fig. 29.24 Large, excavated optic disc with overlying glial tissue and anomalous vascular branching in a patient with papillorenal syndrome.

Other Ophthalmic Features

◆ Poor vision (<20/200)
◆ Visual field defect
◆ Relative afferent pupillary defect

Optic Disc Pit (Fig. 29.25)

Optic disc pit is a congenital gray-white depression usually in the temporal aspect of the optic disc, ⅛ to ⅓ disc diameter in size. Optic disc pit is associated with serous detachment of macula in 30% of cases, resulting in blurred vision and central or paracentral relative scotoma.

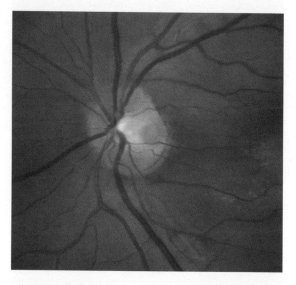

Fig. 29.25   Optic disc pit—grayish depression, measuring approximately ¼ disc diameter, in the temporal aspect of this left optic disc.

Myelinated Nerve Fibers

Myelinated nerve fibers (MNFs) are characterized by patchy, yellow-whitening of the nerve fiber layer with feathery, indistinct borders (**Fig. 29.26**). MNFs represent abnormal myelination of the nerve fibers anterior to the lamina cribrosa of the optic nerve. They are present in 1% of the general population. MNFs may be unilateral or bilateral, single or multiple. They may occur adjacent to the optic disc or elsewhere throughout the posterior pole. The vision is usually normal. Occasionally, MNFs may be associated with enlargement of the physiologic blind spot, subretinal neovascularization, vitreous hemorrhage, and strabismus. Demyelination of MNF may occur during attacks of multiple sclerosis. Small areas of MNF may be mistaken for cotton-wool spots or for astrocytomas.

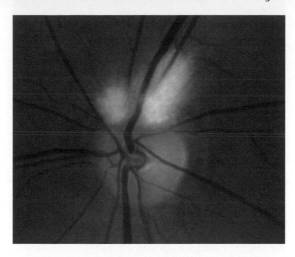

Fig. 29.26   Myelinated nerve fibers—patchy area of whitening of the nerve fibers due to anomalous myelination. The borders are feathery and indistinct.

Glaucomatous Cupping of the Optic Disc

Chronic glaucoma is characterized by an enlarged optic disc cup (**Fig. 29.27**). The neural rim appears thinned, with segmental or diffuse loss of the retinal nerve fiber layer. Superficial splinter hemorrhage may be present on the optic disc. In patients with significant glaucomatous optic disc damage, the cup/disc ratio is usually 0.5 or greater. Other features include:

◆ Inferior notching of the rim
◆ Deviation (banking) of the vessels as they enter the cup

Acute closed-angle glaucoma is associated with optic disc hyperemia with blurring of the margins during the acute attack. In severe cases, cupping of the optic disc, with excavation and pallor, may develop as a late consequence.

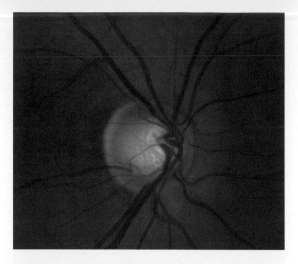

Fig. 29.27 Glaucomatous cupping of the optic disc—increased cup to disc ratio with thinning of the neuronal rim in a patient with glaucoma.

◆ Terson Syndrome

Terson syndrome consists of intraocular hemorrhages associated with acute subarachnoid hemorrhage. Other conditions that can cause a similar ocular event include intracranial and spinal surgery and head trauma. Symptoms include a variable degree of floaters and loss of vision. Intraocular hemorrhages may be present in multiple planes, including intravitreal, subhyaloid, intraretinal, and subretinal spaces (**Fig. 29.28**). Spontaneous improvement occurs in most cases. Vitrectomy may be required for nonclearing vitreous hemorrhage.

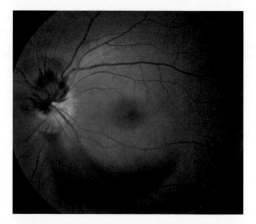

Fig. 29.28 Terson syndrome—intravitreal, disc, retinal, and subretinal hemorrhages in a patient with intracranial hemorrhage due to vascular malformation.

◆ Vascular Malformations

Sturge-Weber Syndrome

Fundus Features

◆ Diffuse choroidal hemangioma—"tomato-catsup" appearance (**Fig. 29.29**)
◆ Localized choroidal hemangioma—yellow-orange, moderately elevated
◆ Exudative retinal detachment

Other Ophthalmic Features

◆ Nevus flammeus (port-wine stain) of the skin and subcutaneous tissue in the distribution of cranial nerve V (**Fig. 29.30**)
◆ Eyelid abnormalities
◆ Congenital glaucoma
◆ Iris heterochromia

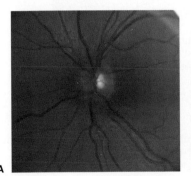
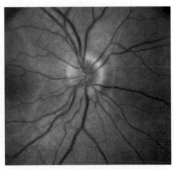

A   **B**

Fig. 29.29 Sturge-Weber syndrome. (**A**) Diffuse choroidal hemangioma with deep-red ("tomato-catsup") appearance of the fundus. (**B**) Normal fellow eye.

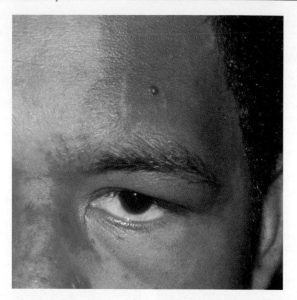

Fig. 29.30   Sturge-Weber syndrome—nevus flammeus (port-wine stain) of the skin in the distribution of the ophthalmic branch of cranial nerve V in a patient with Sturge-Weber syndrome.

Systemic Features

◆ Parieto-occipital leptomeningeal vascular malformation often associated with areas of calcification within the adjacent cerebral cortex
◆ Seizures

Wyburn-Mason Syndrome (Racemose Hemangiomatosis)

Retinal arteriovenous malformation (AVM) associated with intracranial AVM.

Fundus Features (Fig. 29.31)

◆ Retinal AVM
◆ Dilated, tortuous retinal arteries and veins
◆ Arteriolized retinal veins with thick walls
◆ Diminished retinal capillaries
◆ Retinal hemorrhages
◆ Retinal edema and hard exudates

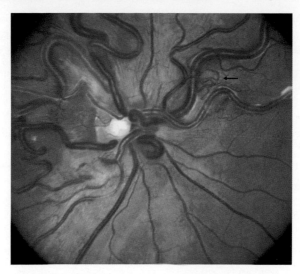

Fig. 29.31 Wyburn-Mason syndrome—retinal arteriovenous malformations (AVMs) (*arrow*) and dilated and tortuous arteries and veins in Wyburn-Mason syndrome. The veins appear "arteriolized" due to the thickening of their walls.

Other Ophthalmic Features

◆ Mild proptosis
◆ Parinaud syndrome
◆ Third, fourth, and sixth cranial nerve palsies

Systemic Features

◆ Hemangiomas
  ○ Midbrain
  ○ Orbit
  ○ Pterygoid fossa
  ○ Mandible
  ○ Maxilla
◆ Intracranial hemorrhage
◆ Seizure
◆ Mental changes
◆ Hemiparesis

Retinal Angiomatosis (von Hippel–Lindau Disease)

Retinal angiomatosis consists of solitary or multiple capillary hemangiomas (hemangioblastomas) of retina or optic disc (**Figs. 29.32 and 29.33**). The condition may be autosomal dominant or sporadic. The abnormal gene is located on chromosome 3. Multiple and bilateral tumors are more likely to have systemic involvement (von Hippel–Lindau disease).

Fundus Features

◆ Pink-red globular, smooth-surfaced vascular tumors
◆ ¼ to 1 disc diameter (DD) in size
◆ Arise from retinal or optic disc vessels
◆ One or more feeder vessels—dilated, tortuous retinal arteries
◆ One or more draining veins—dilated, tortuous retinal veins
◆ Single, multiple, unilateral, or bilateral
◆ Surrounding retinal edema, hard exudates, hemorrhage
◆ Exudative retinal detachment
◆ Vitreoretinal membranes and tractional retinal detachment in severe cases

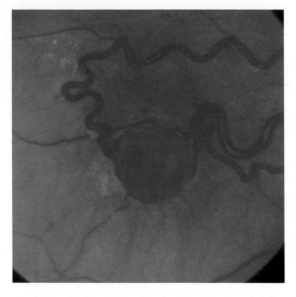

Fig. 29.32   Von Hippel–Lindau disease—retinal capillary hemangioblastoma with feeder and drainage vessels in a patient with intracranial hemangioblastoma.

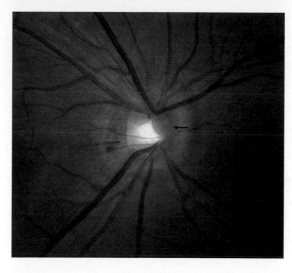

Fig. 29.33 Von Hippel–Lindau disease—small optic disc capillary hemangioblastoma (*arrow*) in a patient with intracranial vascular malformations.

Systemic Features

◆ Cerebellar, spinal hemangioblastoma
◆ Pheochromocytoma
◆ Renal cell carcinoma
◆ Cysts—renal, pancreatic, hepatic, epididymal
◆ Syringomyelia

Dural Arteriovenous Shunt

Cranial arteriovenous shunts are often associated with a history of head trauma. They may be acute and severe (e.g., carotid-cavernous fistula) or chronic and low grade.

Fundus Features (Fig. 29.34)

- Hyperemia of disc
- Optic disc edema
- Disc and retinal hemorrhages
- Dilated, tortuous veins
- Thickened (arteriolized) veins—represent chronicity
- Retinal edema
- Hard exudates
- Cotton-wool spots
- Retinal and optic disc neovascularization
- Vitreous hemorrhage
- Optic atrophy—late feature

Other Ophthalmic Features

- Loss of vision
- Dilated conjunctival vessels/chemosis (**Fig. 29.35**)
- Pulsatile proptosis
- Bruit over upper lid
- Impaired ocular motility
- Elevated intraocular pressure

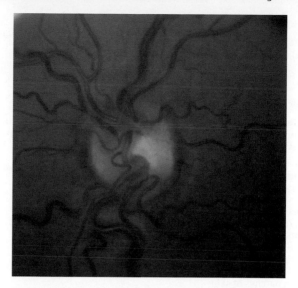

Fig. 29.34 Dural arteriovenous shunt—vascular tortuosity with dilated and arteriolized veins in a patient with low-grade dural arteriovenous shunt.

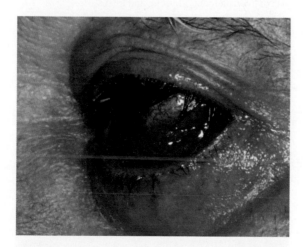

Fig. 29.35 Carotid-cavernous fistula—hemorrhagic chemosis and proptosis in a patient with carotid-cavernous fistula.

◆ Tuberous Sclerosis (Bourneville Syndrome)

Autosomal dominant, chromosome 9

Fundus Features

◆ Characteristic fundus lesion is an astrocytic hamartoma of the retina or optic disc (mulberry tumor) (**Fig. 29.36**). The lesion is a white, semitransparent mulberry-like tumor. Calcification of tumor occurs with age.

Systemic Features

◆ Seizures
◆ Mental deficiency
◆ Adenoma sebaceum (**Fig. 29.37**)
◆ Calcified astrocytic hamartomas of the brain—"brain stones"
◆ Periungual angiofibromas
◆ Café-au-lait spots
◆ Shagreen patches of skin
◆ Ash-leaf spot—depigmented skin macules (**Fig. 29.38**); may also occur on the iris
◆ Cardiac rhabdomyoma, renal cysts, pleural cysts
◆ Cystic bone lesions
◆ Hamartomas of liver, pancreas, thyroid, and testes

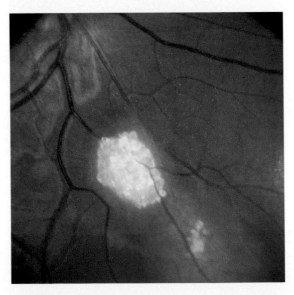

Fig. 29.36   Tuberous sclerosis—astrocytic hamartoma (mulberry tumor) in a patient with tuberous sclerosis.

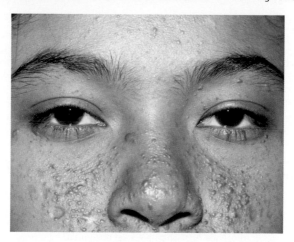

Fig. 29.37 Adenoma sebaceum in the same patient as in **Fig. 29.36**.

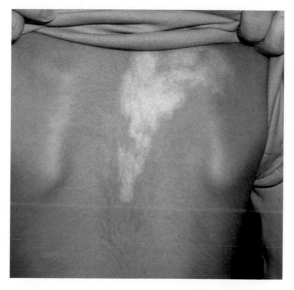

Fig. 29.38 Shagreen skin lesions in a patient with tuberous sclerosis.

Pearls

- The optic disc is located 15 degrees nasal to the fovea. This means that when the patient is looking straight ahead, directing the ophthalmoscope 15 degrees in the horizontal meridian toward the nose will immediately bring the optic disc into view.

- In 80% of individuals, spontaneous venous pulsation is present at the optic disc. The venous pulse is absent in patients with papilledema (intracranial pressure [ICP] >25 cm H_2O). The presence of venous pulsation largely rules out papilledema as the cause of optic disc swelling.

- Optic discs may appear normal in subtle diseases of the optic nerve. In these situations, the presence of a relative afferent pupillary defect and abnormality of color vision are reliable features of optic neuropathy.

- Optic disc drusen are often confused with papilledema. Drusen may be distinguished from papilledema by their refractile, nodular appearance, typical lack of hyperemia and surface microvascular abnormalities (e.g., dilated capillaries and telangiectasis), presence of spontaneous venous pulsation, absence of retinal vascular tortuosity and hemorrhages, and autofluorescence. Deeply buried drusen are more difficult to diagnose. They can be distinguished from papilledema by the presence of venous pulsation, anomalous vascular branching on the disc, and presence of a calcified lesion on B-scan ultrasound or CT scan.

- Anterior optic neuritis can be differentiated from papilledema as follows:

Optic Neuritis	Papilledema
Usually unilateral disc swelling	Usually bilateral
Loss of vision, scotoma	No loss of vision
Abnormal color vision	Color vision unaffected
Relative afferent pupillary defect	Normal pupillary reflex
Pain on eye movement	No pain on eye movement
Mild or no hemorrhage	Often hemorrhage
Mild or no vascular tortuosity	Usually vascular tortuosity

◆ Sickle Cell Hemoglobinopathies

Sickle cell retinopathy is a form of microvascular retinal disease resulting from multiple prior episodes of vascular occlusion. It is usually asymptomatic in the early stages. Patients with more advanced disease may develop visual loss due to vitreous hemorrhage, retinal detachment, and branch or central retinal artery occlusion. Retinal complications occur most frequently in hemoglobin (Hb) SC, followed by Hb SS, and Hb SThal. Hb AS is only rarely associated with retinopathy, usually in conjunction with other diseases, such as diabetes mellitus.

Fundus Features

◆ Increased vascular tortuosity
◆ Abrupt termination of peripheral retinal vessels with "silver-wire" appearances (**Figs. 30.1 and 30.2**)
◆ Retinal vascular sheathing
◆ Peripheral vascular anastomoses
◆ Vascular telangiectasis
◆ "Salmon-patch" retinal hemorrhages (**Figs. 30.3 and 30.4**)
◆ Cotton-wool spots
◆ Central or branch retinal artery occlusion
◆ Abnormal vascular pattern in central macular region
◆ Macular depression sign—abnormal concavity with an irregular central reflection
◆ Macular ischemia, capillary nonperfusion, and enlargement of foveal avascular zone, best seen with fluorescein angiography
◆ Small intraretinal schisis cavities
◆ Iridescent spots (**Fig. 30.5**)
◆ "Black sunburst" chorioretinal scars (**Fig. 30.6**)
◆ "Sea fan" neovascularization—most frequently seen in supratemporal quadrant (**Figs. 30.7 and 30.8**)
◆ Vitreous hemorrhage
◆ Vitreous bands
◆ Retinal detachment—tractional, rhegmatogenous, or combined
◆ Wedge-shaped choroidal infarcts
◆ Choroidal neovascularization—may develop after overly intense laser photocoagulation
◆ Angioid streaks

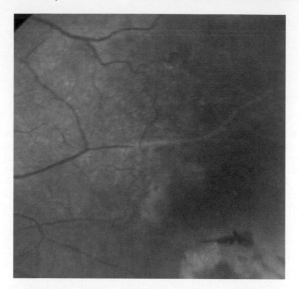

Fig. 30.1 Sickle cell retinopathy—abrupt termination of the peripheral retinal arteries, "silver wire" vessels, peripheral arteriovenous anastomoses, and chorioretinal scar in a patient with sickle cell retinopathy.

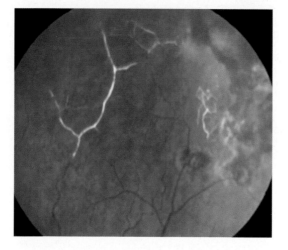

Fig. 30.2 Sickle cell retinopathy—extensive "silver wire" vessels and "black sunburst" chorioretinal scars.

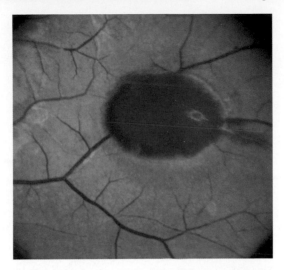

Fig. 30.3 "Salmon-patch" hemorrhage in a patient with sickle cell retinopathy.

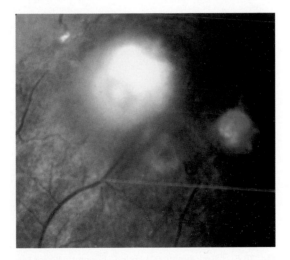

Fig. 30.4 "Salmon-patch" hemorrhages in a patient with sickle cell retinopathy. The smaller "salmon-red" lesion on the right represents recent hemorrhage, and the larger yellowish lesion on the left indicates old, partially hemolyzed hemorrhage.

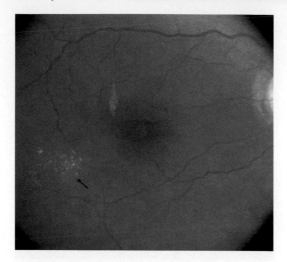

Fig. 30.5 Iridescent spots (*arrow*) in a patient with Hb SC retinopathy. The spots often occur in areas of absorbed hemorrhage.

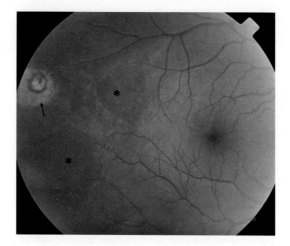

Fig. 30.6 "Black sunburst"—round chorioretinal scar (*arrow*) in a patient with sickle cell disease. There is abrupt termination of the retinal vessels, and the peripheral retina appears featureless due to loss of capillary networks (*asterisks*). Corkscrew vascular tortuosity is present.

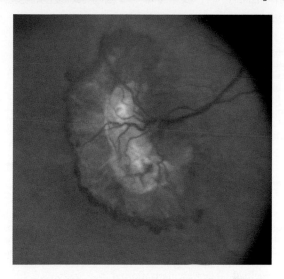

Fig. 30.7 Characteristic "sea fan" neovascularization in a patient with proliferative sickle cell retinopathy.

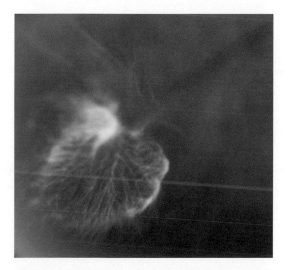

Fig. 30.8 In sickle cell retinopathy, "sea fan" neovascular complexes may spontaneously occlude and undergo "autoinfarction." The occluded vascular network often has a silvery, "ghost vessel" appearance.

Other Ophthalmic Features

◆ Conjunctival comma-shaped vascular changes
◆ Scleral/conjunctival icterus
◆ Iris neovascularization
◆ Proptosis—rare, associated with orbital bone ischemia
◆ Neuro-ophthalmologic
  ◦ Optic disc hemorrhage
  ◦ Ischemic optic neuropathy
  ◦ Cranial nerve palsies
  ◦ Visual field defects

◆ Hyperviscosity Syndrome

Hyperviscosity syndrome is characterized by an increase in the viscosity of blood as a result of increased cellular components, protein concentration, or altered cell morphology. It gives rise to sluggish blood flow through various organs. In the retina, slow blood flow can result in ischemia and secondary changes, including hemorrhage, edema, and neovascularization.

Fundus Features

◆ Retinal hemorrhages (**Fig. 30.9**)
  ◦ Flame-shaped
  ◦ Dot and blot
◆ Microaneurysms
◆ Cotton-wool spots
◆ Dark, tortuous veins
◆ Venous beading
◆ Retinal edema
◆ Serous retinal detachment (**Fig. 30.10**)
◆ Retinal neovascularization—in severe cases
◆ Retinal vein occlusion
◆ Vitreous hemorrhage
◆ Ciliary body cysts—multiple myeloma, Waldenström's macroglobulinemia
◆ Optic disc swelling
  ◦ Papilledema—elevated intracranial pressure
  ◦ Optic disc infiltration (e.g., multiple myeloma, leukemia)
  ◦ Optic disc edema—due to slow flow, retinal vein occlusion

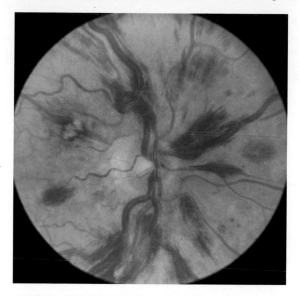

Fig. 30.9 Multiple flame-shaped hemorrhages, few cotton-wool spots, and dot and blot hemorrhages in a patient with hyperviscosity syndrome and Waldenström's macroglobulinemia.

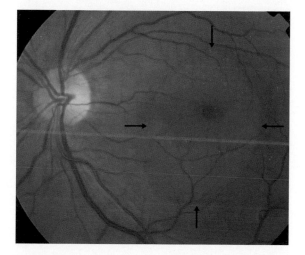

Fig. 30.10 Serous retinal detachment (*arrows*) and fine retinal deposits in a patient with hyperviscosity due to multiple myeloma.

Conditions Associated with Hyperviscosity Syndrome

◆ Polycythemia—primary or secondary
◆ Multiple myeloma
◆ Waldenström's macroglobulinemia
◆ Leukemia
◆ Severe hyperlipidemia
◆ Severe dehydration

◆ Hypercoagulable States

Hypercoagulable states predispose to thrombotic occlusion of blood vessels. In the eye this may manifest as:

◆ Central or branch retinal vein occlusion (**Fig. 30.11**)
◆ Central or branch retinal artery occlusion
◆ Ophthalmic artery occlusion
◆ Choroidal infarcts

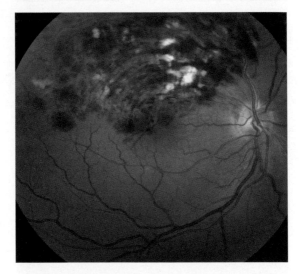

Fig. 30.11   Multiple retinal hemorrhages and cotton-wool spots in a patient with branch retinal vein occlusion associated with anticardiolipin antibody syndrome.

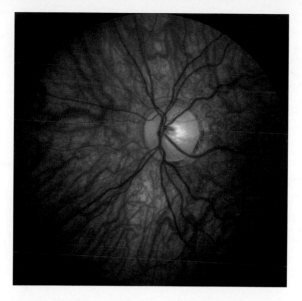

Fig. 33.1 Albinism—diffusely hypopigmented fundus with visible choroidal vasculature.

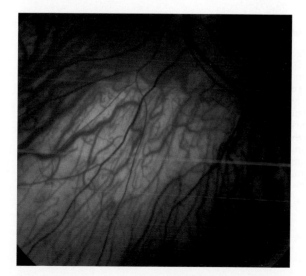

Fig. 33.2 Albinism—hypopigmented (blond) peripheral fundus in a patient with albinism. Choroidal vasculature is distinctly visible due to diminished pigment in the retinal pigment epithelium and choriocapillary layer.

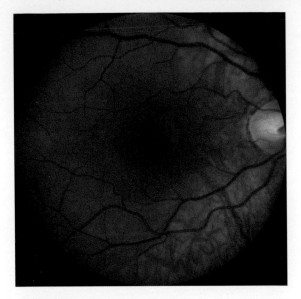

Fig. 33.3 Abnormal (missing) foveal light reflex with absence of foveal pit, hypopigmented fundus, and visible choroidal vessels in a patient with albinism.

Other Ophthalmic Features

◆ Decreased vision
◆ Photophobia
◆ Abnormal color vision
◆ Impaired binocular function and stereopsis
◆ Refractive error
◆ Light-colored iris
◆ Iris transillumination (**Fig. 33.4**)
◆ Pink light reflex through undilated pupil
◆ Strabismus
◆ Nystagmus
◆ Abnormal chiasmal decussation

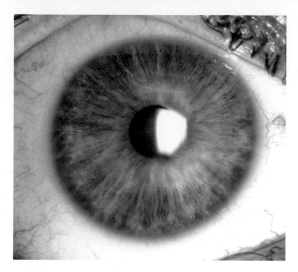

Fig. 33.4 Peripheral iris transillumination in a patient with ocular albinism.

Systemic Features

◆ Fair skin
◆ Blond hair
◆ Bleeding disorder
  ∘ Hermansky-Pudlak syndrome is an autosomal recessive disorder characterized by platelet dysfunction and albinism. Other features include pulmonary fibrosis, colitis, and renal failure. It occurs most frequently in individuals of Puerto Rican descent.
◆ Immune deficiency
  ∘ Chediak-Higashi syndrome is an autosomal recessive disorder affecting white blood cells, causing susceptibility to frequent infections and lymphoma. Features include patchy albinism, frequent infections, peripheral neuropathy, and mental retardation.

◆ Oculodermal Melanocytosis

Oculodermal melanocytosis (ODM) is a congenital melanocytic hyperpigmentation of the ocular tissue and face, particularly in the distribution of the ophthalmic and maxillary divisions of the fifth cranial nerve. Ninety percent of cases are unilateral. Synonyms for ODM include ocular melanocytosis, melanosis oculi, melanosis bulbi, and nevus of Ota.

Fundus Features

- Choroidal hyperpigmentation—unilateral, patchy
- Optic disc pigmentation—rare
- Choroidal melanoma—Individuals with ODM have increased risk of developing uveal melanoma. ODM occurs more commonly in darkly pigmented individuals, who have less risk of developing choroidal melanoma compared with light-skinned individuals.

Other Ophthalmic Features

- Eyelid and facial skin hyperpigmentation (**Fig. 33.5**)
- Conjunctival hyperpigmentation
- Episcleral and scleral pigmentation (**Fig. 33.6**)—slate-gray patchy pigmentation
- Iris hyperpigmentation
- Glaucoma
- Cataract
- Uveitis
- Orbital melanoma
- Hyperpigmentation of the nasal or buccal mucosa

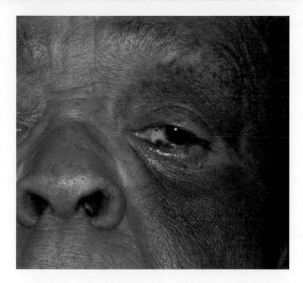

Fig. 33.5 Oculodermal melanocytosis (ODM)—congenital hyperpigmentation of the skin in the distribution of the ophthalmic and maxillary nerves.

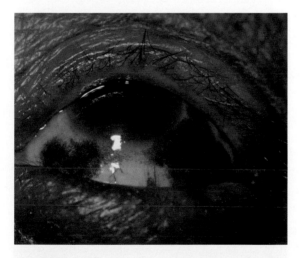

Fig. 33.6 Oculodermal melanocytosis (ODM)—conjunctival, episcleral, and scleral hyperpigmentation in the same patient as in **Fig. 33.5**.

◆ Incontinentia Pigmenti (Bloch-Sulzberger Syndrome)

Incontinentia pigmenti is an X-linked dominant ectodermal dysplasia, affecting skin, hair, teeth, central nervous system, and eyes.

Fundus Features

◆ Avascular peripheral retina (**Fig. 33.7**)
◆ Retinal telangiectasis
◆ Peripheral retinal arteriovenous anastomoses (**Fig. 33.8**)—irregular, tortuous vessels at the junction of vascularized and avascular retina
◆ Retinal arteriolar aneurysms
◆ Foveal distortion secondary to foveal avascularity (**Fig. 33.9**)
◆ Retinal hemorrhage
◆ Retinal neovascularization
◆ Preretinal fibrosis
◆ "Dragging" of retinal vessels (**Fig. 33.10**)
◆ Persistent fetal vasculature
◆ Exudative retinal detachment
◆ Tractional retinal detachment
◆ Rhegmatogenous retinal detachment
◆ Vitreous hemorrhage
◆ Retinal pigment epithelial abnormalities
◆ Optic atrophy

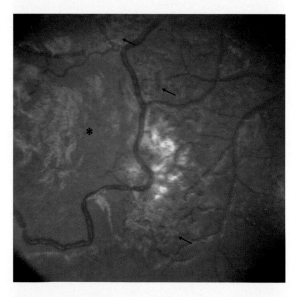

Fig. 33.7   Incontinentia pigmenti—avascular peripheral retina (*asterisk*) and retinal telangiectasis (*arrows*).

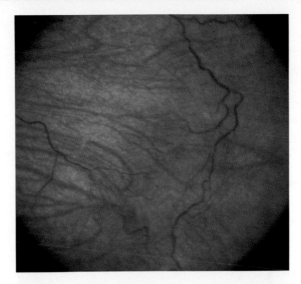

Fig. 33.8 Incontinentia pigmenti—avascular peripheral retina with arteriovenous anastomoses and telangiectasis.

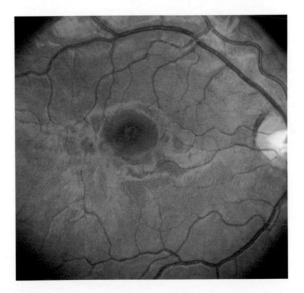

Fig. 33.9 Abnormal foveal reflex and distortion in a patient with incontinentia pigmenti.

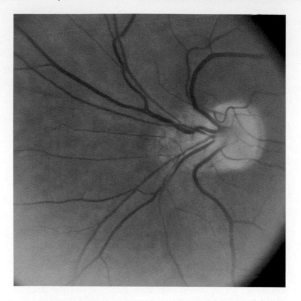

Fig. 33.10   Incontinentia pigmenti—"dragging" of the retinal vessels and the optic disc.

Other Ophthalmic Features

- Diminished vision
- Conjunctival pigmentation
- Strabismus
- Nystagmus
- Cataract
- Cortical blindness
- Phthisis—end stage

Systemic Features

◆ Skin (**Fig. 33.11**)
  ◦ Erythematous macules, papules, vesicles, and bullae
  ◦ Verrucous lesions
  ◦ Hyperpigmented and hypopigmented whorls and streaks
  ◦ Alopecia
◆ Hypodontia
◆ Neurologic
  ◦ Cerebral edema, hemorrhage, and cyst formation
  ◦ Cerebral atrophy
  ◦ Gyrate dysplasia
  ◦ Cortical blindness
◆ Epilepsy

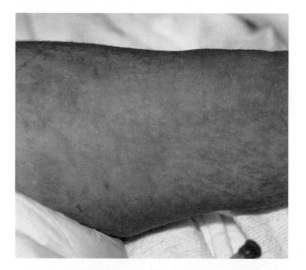

Fig. 33.11   Verrucous skin lesions in a patient with incontinentia pigmenti.

◆ Pseudoxanthoma Elasticum

Pseudoxanthoma elasticum affects the skin and eye, as well as the cardiovascular and gastrointestinal systems. It is characterized by production of abnormal elastic fibers and secondary tissue calcification.

Fundus Features

◆ Angioid streaks
  ◦ Angioid streaks are bilateral, irregular linear subretinal lesions that can incompletely encircle the optic disc and radiate peripherally (**Fig. 33.12**). Depending on chronicity and race, the color varies from yellow-white to red-brown to dark brown. Angioid streaks represent cracks in Bruch's membrane.
◆ Peau d'orange changes—mottled appearance of fundus (**Fig. 33.13**)
◆ Choroidal neovascularization
◆ Subretinal hemorrhage
◆ Multiple, punched-out yellowish atrophic peripheral lesions
◆ Intraretinal crystal deposition
◆ Reticular macular pigmentation
◆ Optic disc drusen
◆ Myopic degeneration
◆ Retinal detachment

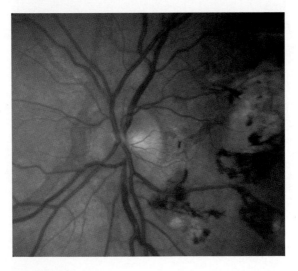

Fig. 33.12 Angioid streaks—dark red subretinal bands of angioid streaks surrounding the optic disc and radiating toward the periphery in a patient with pseudoxanthoma elasticum. Subretinal scars, indicating prior episodes of choroidal neovascularization, are also present.

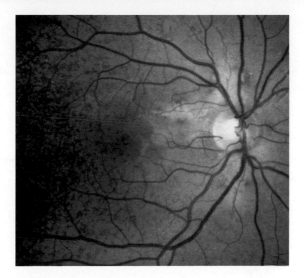

Fig. 33.13   Peau d'orange pigmentary changes of the fundus and subtle subretinal bands of angioid streaks in a patient with pseudoxanthoma elasticum.

Other Ophthalmic Features

◆ High myopia
◆ Subluxation of lens

Systemic Features

◆ Autosomal recessive inheritance (rarely dominant)
◆ Skin (**Fig. 33.14**)
  ◦ Redundant, waxy, yellow, papule-like lesions ("plucked chicken") on neck, face, oral mucosa, axilla, abdomen, and inguinal region
  ◦ Soft tissue calcification
◆ Cardiovascular
  ◦ Intracranial aneurysms
  ◦ Aortic aneurysm
  ◦ Heart valve abnormality
  ◦ Peripheral vascular disease
◆ Gastrointestinal ulceration and hemorrhage
◆ Musculoskeletal
  ◦ Hyperextensible joints
  ◦ Ligamentous calcification
◆ Neurologic
  ◦ Intracerebral and subarachnoid hemorrhage
  ◦ Intracerebral calcification
  ◦ Cerebral atrophy

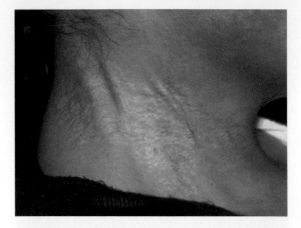

Fig. 33.14   Waxy, yellow, papule-like skin lesions ("plucked chicken") on the neck of a patient with pseudoxanthoma elasticum.

◆ Ehlers-Danlos Syndrome

Ehlers-Danlos syndrome (EDS) is a heterogeneous group of heritable connective tissue disorders. Most cases have autosomal dominant inheritance. The classic form of EDS is characterized by skin hyperextensibility with atrophic scars, joint hypermobility, and general tissue fragility.

Fundus Features

- ◆ Angioid streaks
- ◆ Choroidal neovascularization
- ◆ Subretinal hemorrhage
- ◆ Retinal detachment
- ◆ Myopic degeneration
- ◆ Pigment abnormalities

Other Ophthalmic Features

- ◆ Myopia, astigmatism
- ◆ Amblyopia
- ◆ Eyelid laxity
- ◆ Epicanthal folds
- ◆ Thin, blue sclera
- ◆ Thin cornea
- ◆ Keratoconus, keratoglobus
- ◆ Glaucoma
- ◆ Lens dislocation
- ◆ Strabismus

Systemic Features

◆ Skin laxity
◆ Skin fragility and poor wound healing
◆ "Cigarette paper" scarring of skin
◆ Hypermobile joints
◆ Recurrent joint dislocations
◆ Scoliosis
◆ Muscle hypotony
◆ Mitral valve prolapse
◆ Arterial aneurysms
◆ Pneumothorax
◆ Polycystic kidneys
◆ Platelet aggregation abnormalities
◆ Maldeveloped teeth

Pearls

- Autoimmune disorders that cause vitiligo may also affect the retinal pigment epithelium, resulting in patchy areas of chorioretinal depigmentation. These lesions are not visually significant.

- Uveitic conditions such as Vogt-Koyanagi-Harada syndrome and sympathetic ophthalmia may be associated with vitiligo, hair loss, and whitening of hair or eyelashes.

◆ Retinal Vasculitis

Retinal vasculitis can affect retinal arteries, veins, or both. It can occur in isolation or in association with an underlying systemic disease. The inflammatory process may cause occlusion of small or major retinal vessels, giving rise to visual loss. Initially, the condition may be asymptomatic. Symptoms include painless loss of vision, scotomas, and floaters.

Fundus Features

◆ Venous or arterial sheathing (**Figs. 34.1, 34.2, and 34.3**)
◆ Attenuated or occluded arterioles and venules
◆ Retinal hemorrhages
◆ Microaneurysms
◆ Cotton-wool spots
◆ Edema
◆ Hard exudates
◆ Telangiectasis
◆ Retinal neovascularization
◆ Retinal necrosis—pale creamy retina; represents severe, acute retinal vasculitis
◆ Vitreous hemorrhage
◆ Tractional retinal detachment
◆ Rhegmatogenous retinal detachment

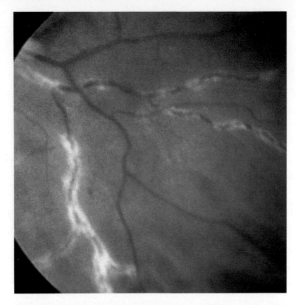

Fig. 34.1 Sheathing of retinal artery characteristic of retinal vasculitis.

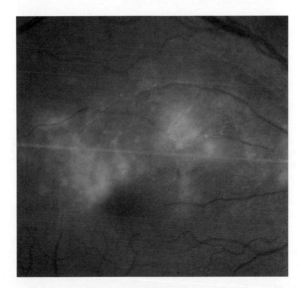

Fig. 34.2 Segmental sheathing of small retinal arteries and patchy areas of retinitis in a patient with herpes retinitis.

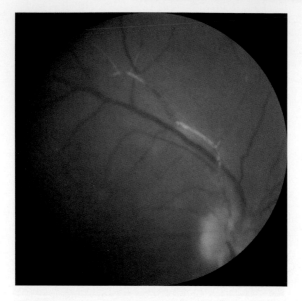

Fig. 34.3   Retinal vasculitis with sheathing of artery and optic neuropathy in a patient with acute retinal necrosis.

Conditions Associated with Retinal Vasculitis

- Primary idiopathic retinal vasculitis (also termed Eales disease)
- Systemic lupus erythematosus (SLE)
- Vasculitides
  - Giant cell arteritis
  - Wegener granulomatosis
  - Polyarteritis nodosa
  - Churg-Strauss angiitis
  - Henoch-Schönlein purpura
  - Takayasu arteritis
- Sarcoidosis
- Behçet disease
- Inflammatory bowel disease
- Multiple sclerosis
- Radiation therapy
- Infectious diseases
  - Syphilis
  - Tuberculosis
  - Lyme disease
  - Cat-scratch disease
  - Toxoplasmosis
  - Viral—cytomegalovirus, herpes simplex, herpes zoster
- Ocular
  - Pars planitis
  - Bird-shot chorioretinopathy
  - Other forms of chorioretinitis may be associated with segmental retinal vasculitis.

◆ Systemic Lupus Erythematosus (Fig. 34.4)

SLE is a multisystem autoimmune disorder characterized by polyarthritis, skin lesions, systemic vasculitis, renal disease, neurologic involvement, pericarditis, pleuritis, lymphadenopathy, hepatitis, and anemia.

Fundus Features

- ◆ Cotton-wool spots
- ◆ Retinal hemorrhages
- ◆ Microaneurysms
- ◆ Retinal vasculitis—vascular sheathing
- ◆ Retinal vascular occlusion
- ◆ Retinal neovascularization
- ◆ Vitreous hemorrhage
- ◆ Serous/exudative retinal detachment
- ◆ Choroiditis—patchy
- ◆ Choroidal infarction
- ◆ Choroidal neovascularization
- ◆ Choroidal scar
- ◆ Optic neuritis
- ◆ SLE-induced hypertensive retinopathy
- ◆ Chloroquine/hydroxychloroquine maculopathy

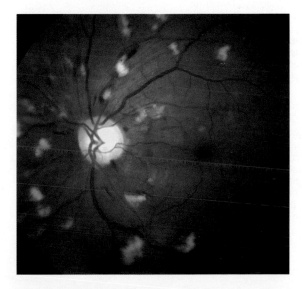

Fig. 34.4 Multiple cotton-wool spots and flame-shaped hemorrhages indicating retinal microvasculopathy in systemic lupus erythematosus.

Other Ophthalmic Features

◆ Keratoconjunctivitis sicca
◆ Scleritis
◆ Keratitis
◆ Uveitis

◆ Wegener Granulomatosis

Wegener granulomatosis is a vasculitis of small and medium-sized vessels that has many extravascular manifestations. Involvement of the paranasal sinuses, lower airways, kidneys, and eyes is characteristic. Inflammatory pseudotumors may form in many tissues, including the lungs and orbit. Most patients are positive for cytoplasmic-staining antineutrophil cytoplasmic antibody (C-ANCA). Perinuclear-staining antineutrophil cytoplasmic antibody (P-ANCA) may also be positive.

Fundus Features

◆ Cotton-wool spots
◆ Retinal hemorrhages
◆ Retinal vasculitis—vascular sheathing
◆ Retinal vascular occlusion
◆ Retinal neovascularization
◆ Vitreous hemorrhage
◆ Serous/exudative retinal detachment
◆ Retinitis
◆ Ischemic optic neuropathy—pale swelling of the optic disc
◆ Optic atrophy—pale disc

Other Ophthalmic Features

◆ Visual loss
◆ Visual field abnormalities
◆ Scleritis (**Fig. 34.5**)
◆ Keratitis
◆ Uveitis
◆ Proptosis
◆ Orbital inflammation
◆ Cranial nerve palsies

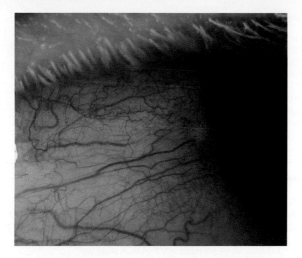

Fig. 34.5 Congestion of scleral and episcleral blood vessels indicating scleritis in Wegener granulomatosis. Patchy corneal stromal infiltrates are also present.

◆ Polyarteritis Nodosa

Polyarteritis nodosa is characterized by a necrotizing vasculitis of small and medium-sized arteries. Lesions are often present at the arterial branch points and can lead to stenosis, aneurysm formation, hemorrhage, thrombosis, and infarction. Kidneys, gastrointestinal tract, and the peripheral and central nervous systems are often affected. Most patients test positive for P-ANCA.

Fundus Features

- ◆ Retinal hemorrhages
- ◆ Cotton-wool spots
- ◆ Retinal vasculitis—vascular sheathing
- ◆ Retinal vascular occlusion
- ◆ Retinal neovascularization
- ◆ Vitreous hemorrhage
- ◆ Serous retinal detachment
- ◆ Hypertensive retinopathy
- ◆ Choroidal ischemia
- ◆ Ischemic optic neuropathy—pale swelling of the optic disc
- ◆ Optic atrophy—pale disc
- ◆ Acute multifocal placoid pigment epitheliopathy/choroidopathy

Other Ophthalmic Features

◆ Visual loss
◆ Visual field abnormalities
◆ Scleritis
◆ Keratitis
◆ Uveitis
◆ Cogan syndrome—interstitial keratitis, hearing loss, vasculitis
◆ Cranial nerve palsies
◆ Optic neuropathy

◆ Churg-Strauss Syndrome

Churg-Strauss syndrome (allergic granulomatosis) is a vasculitis affecting small and medium-sized vessels. Systemic features include chronic asthma, pulmonary infiltrates, vasculitis, eosinophilia, skin lesions, and gastrointestinal and neurologic manifestations. Most patients are P-ANCA positive.

Fundus Features

◆ Retinal hemorrhage
◆ Retinal vasculitis—vascular sheathing
◆ Retinal vascular occlusion
◆ Retinal neovascularization
◆ Hypertensive retinopathy
◆ Serous retinal detachment
◆ Ischemic optic neuropathy—pale swelling of the optic disc
◆ Optic atrophy—pale disc
◆ Choroidal ischemia

Other Ophthalmic Features

◆ Visual loss
◆ Visual field abnormalities
◆ Conjunctival granulomas
◆ Scleritis
◆ Keratitis
◆ Uveitis
◆ Cranial nerve palsies

◆ Giant Cell Arteritis

Giant cell arteritis (GCA), also known as temporal arteritis, is characterized by a granulomatous inflammation of medium-sized arteries, particularly branches of the carotid
artery. GCA affects patients older than 50 years and occurs more frequently in females.
Features include headaches, scalp and temple area tenderness, fatigue, weight loss,
low-grade fever, anemia, arthralgia and stiffness (shoulders and hips), jaw claudica-
tions, angina, vision loss, and other ocular manifestations. Involvement of the aorta
and its branches may give rise to additional symptoms. Erythrocyte sedimentation
rate is significantly elevated in 90% of patients at the time of presentation.

Fundus Features

- ◆ Ischemic optic neuropathy—pale swelling of optic disc, splinter hemorrhages at
  the margin, and late optic atrophy
- ◆ Central retinal artery occlusion
- ◆ Ophthalmic artery occlusion
- ◆ Retinal neovascularization
- ◆ Iris neovascularization
- ◆ Choroidal ischemia/infarct
- ◆ Serous retinal detachment—due to choroidal ischemia
- ◆ Choroidal scar
- ◆ Optic atrophy—pale disc; late feature

Other Ophthalmic Features

- ◆ Loss of vision
- ◆ Impaired color vision
- ◆ Visual field defects
- ◆ Diplopia
- ◆ Relative afferent pupillary defect (RAPD)
- ◆ Cranial nerve palsies
- ◆ Extraocular muscle palsy

◆ Relapsing Polychondritis

Relapsing polychondritis is characterized by recurrent episodes of inflammation
in the cartilage of various tissues, including joints, nose ("saddle nose" deformity),
larynx, bronchi, external ear ("cauliflower ear"), middle and inner ear, heart, and
the aorta. Other features include vasculitis, glomerulonephritis, stroke, aseptic
meningitis, skin lesions, orogenital ulcers, and superficial thrombophlebitis. Ocular manifestations occur in 60% of patients.

Fundus Features

◆ Retinal hemorrhages
◆ Cotton-wool spots
◆ Retinal vasculitis—vascular sheathing
◆ Retinal vascular occlusion
◆ Serous retinal detachment
◆ Ischemic optic neuropathy—pale swelling of the optic disc
◆ Pale disc—optic atrophy

Other Ophthalmic Features

◆ Scleritis
◆ Keratitis
◆ Corneal "melt"
◆ Conjunctivitis
◆ Uveitis
◆ Inflammation of eyelids—tarsitis
◆ Orbital pseudotumor
◆ Cranial nerve palsies

◆ Rheumatoid Arthritis

Rheumatoid arthritis (RA) is a systemic disease characterized by progressive, symmetrical, inflammatory polyarthritis and constitutional features. Synovial membrane inflammation and destructive lesions of surrounding cartilage and bone are hallmarks. Rheumatoid factor is positive in 75% of patients with RA. There is an association between human leukocyte antigen (HLA) DR4 and RA.

Fundus Features

Retinal involvement by RA is rare and is usually the result of secondary conditions such as vasculitis and anemia.

◆ Retinal hemorrhages
◆ Cotton-wool spots
◆ Retinal edema
◆ Retinal vascular sheathing—representing vasculitis
◆ Serous retinal detachment—secondary to posterior scleritis
◆ Choroidal effusion—secondary to posterior scleritis
◆ Toxic maculopathy—"bull's-eye" maculopathy from hydroxychloroquine toxicity
◆ Keratoconjunctivitis sicca
◆ Episcleritis
◆ Scleritis
◆ Scleral ectasia (**Fig. 34.6**)
◆ Keratitis—corneal "melt"
◆ Uveitis—rare

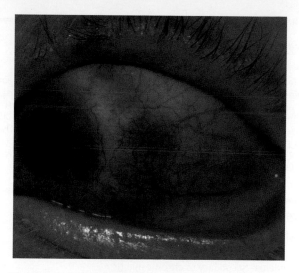

Fig. 34.6 Scleral thinning (ectasia) in a patient with rheumatoid arthritis. The darker color of the uveal tissue is transmitted through the sclera, resulting in a bluish appearance in the area of thinning.

Systemic Features

- Articular
  - Morning stiffness
  - "Gelling"—improvement of joint stiffness with use
  - Symmetric joint swelling
  - Joint subluxation—ulnar deviation, swan-neck deformity of proximal interphalangeal joints, atlantoaxial subluxation
  - Erosion of cartilage and bone
  - Inflammatory synovial fluid
  - Carpal tunnel syndrome
  - Baker's cyst—rupture of synovial fluid from the knee into the calf
  - Most commonly involved joints
    - Proximal interphalangeal joints
    - Metacarpophalangeal joints
    - Wrists
    - Small joints of feet, ankle
    - Cervical spine
    - Other—elbow, hips, shoulder
- Rheumatoid nodules—subcutaneous, pulmonary, myocardial, scleral
- Constitutional—fever, malaise, weight loss
- Pleuritis, pleural effusion, interstitial lung disease
- Pericarditis, pericardial effusion, heart block, myocardial infarction
- Vasculitis
- Stroke
- Raynaud's phenomenon
- Glomerulonephritis
- Polyneuropathy, cervical myelopathy
- Anemia, leukopenia, lymphadenopathy
- Leg ulcers
- Felty syndrome—splenomegaly, leukopenia, and RA
- Secondary amyloidosis

◆ Ankylosing Spondylitis

Systemic features of ankylosing spondylitis include chronic low back pain, fusion of axial skeleton, sacroiliitis, arthritis of large joints and ribs, scoliosis, limited chest movement, restrictive lung disease, apical pulmonary fibrosis, aortitis, aortic valve incompetence, and heart block. Ocular complications occur in 25% of patients. Onset of symptoms is in the second and third decades of life. Over 90% of Caucasian patients with ankylosing spondylitis are HLA-B27 positive (compared with 7% of general population). Spinal x-rays characteristically show "bamboo spine" and sacroiliac joint abnormalities.

Fundus Features

Retina is rarely affected by ankylosing spondylitis.

◆ Vitritis
◆ Macular edema—secondary to chronic uveitis
◆ Serous retinal detachment—secondary to posterior scleritis

Other Ophthalmic Features

◆ Anterior uveitis—recurrent, chronic
◆ Secondary glaucoma
◆ Secondary cataract
◆ Episcleritis and scleritis

◆ Reiter Syndrome

Reiter syndrome includes the triad of arthritis, urethritis, and conjunctivitis. Seventy-five percent of patients are HLA-B27 positive. Other features include plantar fasciitis, calcaneal periostitis, circinate balanitis, prostatitis, cervicitis, keratoderma blenorrhagicum, aphthous mouth ulcers, nail abnormalities, pericarditis, myocarditis, aortitis, fever, and weight loss.

Ophthalmic Features

◆ Conjunctivitis—Noninfectious conjunctivitis is present in 60% of patients.
◆ Keratitis
◆ Anterior uveitis—present in 20%
◆ Posterior uveitis—rare
◆ Retinal vasculitis—rare
◆ Optic neuropathy—rare

◆ Sjögren Syndrome

Primary Sjögren syndrome is an autoimmune inflammatory condition character-ized by dry mouth and dry eyes. Secondary Sjögren syndrome is the triad of dry mouth, dry eyes, and an underlying systemic connective tissue disease.

Fundus Features

Fundus changes are rarely seen in primary Sjögren syndrome, but the associated connective tissue disease of secondary Sjögren syndrome may also result in retinal changes that are characteristic of the underlying disease.

Other Ophthalmic Features

◆ Dry-eye symptoms
◆ Mucoid discharge
◆ Chronic low-grade conjunctivitis
◆ Conjunctival scarring
◆ Conjunctival keratinization
◆ Keratitis
◆ Corneal scarring
◆ Corneal vascularization
◆ Corneal "melt"
◆ Filamentary keratoconjunctivitis

◆ Juvenile Spondyloarthropathy (Juvenile Rheumatoid Arthritis)

Subtypes of juvenile spondyloarthropathy include the following:

◆ Systemic onset (Still disease)—affects girls and boys equally. It is antinuclear an-tibody (ANA) and rheumatoid factor (RF) negative. Features include fever, rash, lymphadenopathy, hepatitis, splenomegaly, serositis, polyarthritis, leukocyto-sis, and elevated sedimentation rate.
◆ Rheumatoid factor positive juvenile rheumatoid arthritis—resembles adult RA. Girls are more frequently affected than boys.
◆ Polyarticular juvenile arthritis—RF negative; mild fever, anemia, growth retar-dation
◆ Early-onset pauciarticular juvenile arthritis—ANA positive (50%), RF negative. Girls are more frequently affected than boys. High risk of ocular involvement (50%).
◆ Late-onset pauciarticular juvenile arthritis—ANA negative, RF negative. Pre-dominantly affects boys. May resemble ankylosing spondylitis.

Fundus Features

◆ Macular edema—secondary to chronic anterior uveitis
◆ Intermediate uveitis
◆ Peripheral vitreous and chorioretinal infiltrates
◆ Epiretinal membrane

Other Ophthalmic Features

◆ Anterior uveitis—chronic, recurrent
◆ Secondary glaucoma
◆ Secondary cataract
◆ Band-shaped keratopathy

◆ Behçet Syndrome

Behçet syndrome is a multisystem disease characterized by the triad of oral ulcers, genital ulcers, and uveitis. Other features include arthritis, migratory superficial thrombophlebitis, major vessel thrombosis, arterial aneurysms, gastrointestinal ulceration, erythema nodosum, pyoderma, dermatographia, and positive patergy test. Central nervous system (CNS) abnormalities, including brainstem abnormalities, meningoencephalitis, and dural sinus thrombosis, are serious complications. Behçet syndrome is associated with HLA-B51.

Fundus Features (Fig. 34.7)

◆ Retinal hemorrhages
◆ Retinal infiltrates
◆ Cotton-wool spots
◆ Perivascular sheathing
◆ Macular edema
◆ Retinal artery occlusion
◆ Retinal vein occlusion
◆ Retinal inflammatory infiltrates
◆ Retinal neovascularization
◆ Optic neuropathy
◆ Vitritis
◆ Vitreous hemorrhage

Other Ophthalmic Features

◆ Anterior uveitis
◆ Sterile hypopyon

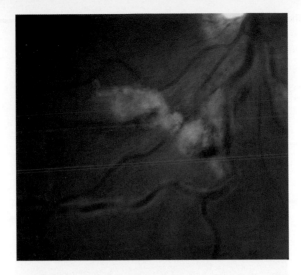

Fig. 34.7 Behçet syndrome—perivenous sheathing, retinal hemorrhages, and cotton-wool spots.

◆ Vogt-Koyanagi-Harada Syndrome

Vogt-Koyanagi-Harada (VKH) syndrome is a granulomatous inflammatory disease affecting eyes, meninges, and skin. It is characterized by bilateral anterior and posterior uveitis, serous retinal detachments, meningeal irritation, hearing loss, and vitiligo. Other nonocular features include fever, malaise, nausea, headaches, photophobia, neck rigidity, vertigo, tinnitus, dysacusia, and hair loss. VKH primarily affects adults in the third to sixth decades of life. It occurs more frequently in Asians and darkly pigmented races.

Fundus Features

◆ Serous retinal detachment (**Fig. 34.8**)
◆ Retinal edema
◆ Hard exudates
◆ Focal subretinal/choroidal inflammatory infiltrates—"Dalen-Fuchs" nodules are yellow-white round subretinal lesions with ill-defined borders.
◆ Patchy, or diffuse subretinal/choroidal inflammatory infiltrates
◆ Retinal vascular sheathing
◆ Optic disc hyperemia and edema
◆ Vitritis
◆ Late features
  ○ Retinal pigment epithelium (RPE) mottling and diffuse atrophy ("sunset glow" fundus) (**Fig. 34.9**)
  ○ Focal or diffuse pigmented chorioretinal scars
  ○ Choroidal neovascularization (CNV)—may cause subretinal hemorrhage and visual loss
  ○ Optic atrophy—pale optic disc
  ○ Vascular sheathing
  ○ Ghost vessels

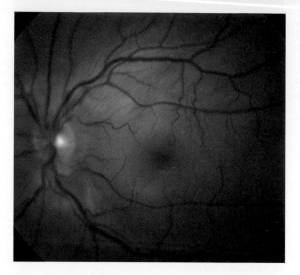

Fig. 34.8 Retinal folds in an area of serous retinal detachment, and optic disc hyperemia in a 24-year-old woman with Vogt-Koyanagi-Harada syndrome.

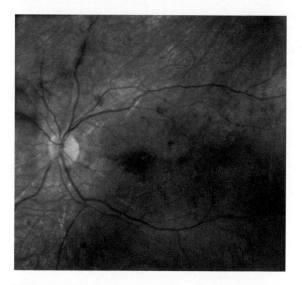

Fig. 34.9 "Sunset-glow" fundus with diffuse retinal pigment epithelial mottling and atrophy and pigment clumping in a patient with chronic Vogt-Koyanagi-Harada syndrome and resolved serous retinal detachment.

Other Ophthalmic Features

◆ Blurred vision
◆ Poliosis—whitening of the eye lashes (**Fig. 34.10**)
◆ Perilimbal vitiligo—Sugiura sign
◆ Anterior uveitis
◆ Keratic precipitates (KPs)—"Mutton-fat" KPs represent granulomatous uveitis
◆ Irregular pupil—due to posterior synechiae
◆ Iris nodules
◆ Secondary glaucoma
◆ Secondary cataract
◆ Secondary ocular hypotony

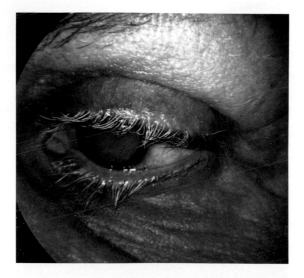

Fig. 34.10   Poliosis—whitening of the eyelashes in Vogt-Koy-anagi-Harada syndrome.

◆ Marfan Syndrome

Marfan syndrome is an autosomal dominant connective tissue disorder with a defect in the fibrillin 1 gene on chromosome 15. Features of Marfan syndrome include tall stature, arachnodactyly, joint laxity, high-arched palate, pectus deformities, heart valve disease, cardiac arrhythmias, aortic aneurysm, pulmonary cysts, spontaneous pneumothorax, and ocular abnormalities.

Fundus Features

◆ Myopic degeneration
◆ Lattice retinal degeneration
◆ Retinal detachment

Other Ophthalmic Features

◆ High myopia
◆ Ectopia lentis—subluxation of lens, usually bilateral and in supratemporal direction (**Fig. 34.11**)
◆ Iridodonesis
◆ Cataract
◆ Glaucoma
◆ Keratoconus

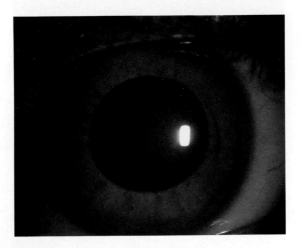

Fig. 34.11   Subluxation of the crystalline lens in a 32-year-old woman with Marfan syndrome.

◆ Stickler Syndrome

Stickler syndrome is an autosomal dominant connective tissue disorder with mutation in the type II procollagen gene. It is characterized by progressive arthropathy, epiphyseal dysplasia, midfacial flattening, hearing loss, cleft palate, high myopia, and retinal detachment.

Fundus Features

- ◆ Lattice retinal degeneration—often pigmented, paravascular, posteriorly located and with radial orientation
- ◆ Paravascular pigmentation
- ◆ Multiple, posterior retinal tears
- ◆ Giant retinal tear
- ◆ Retinal detachment
- ◆ Peripheral vascular sheathing
- ◆ Choroidal hypopigmentation
- ◆ Premature vitreous syneresis
- ◆ Optically empty spaces in the vitreous cavity
- ◆ Vitreous veils

Other Ophthalmic Features

- ◆ High myopia
- ◆ Cataract
- ◆ Glaucoma

◆ Chloroquine and Hydroxychloroquine Maculopathy

Chloroquine and hydroxychloroquine maculopathy is discussed in the section on Hydroxychloroquine (Plaquenil)/Chloroquine in Chapter 39.

> **Pearls**
>
> - Diagnosis of retinal vasculitis is based on the ophthalmoscopic finding of vascular sheathing and fundus fluorescein angiographic findings of segmental staining and leakage of the retinal vessels.

35 Oncology

◆ Choroidal Nevus

Choroidal nevus is the most common pigmented lesion of the fundus. It is present in 30% of the general population and usually has no visual implications unless secondary problems, such as choroidal neovascularization, occur. Choroidal nevi may be solitary, multiple, unilateral, or bilateral. Malignant transformation may occur, but is uncommon.

Fundus Features

- ◆ Flat, pigmented (gray-brown), subretinal lesions of varying size (**Fig. 35.1**)
  - ∘ Minimally thickened—<2 mm
  - ∘ Usually <5 mm (<3 disc diameters [DD]) in diameter
- ◆ Overlying retinal vessels
- ◆ Overlying drusen—suggestive of a chronic, benign lesion
- ◆ May become depigmented with time
- ◆ Retinal pigment epithelial atrophy/hypertrophy
- ◆ Choroidal neovascularization—uncommon
- ◆ Marked enlargement is rare

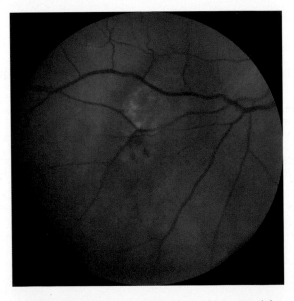

Fig. 35.1 Choroidal nevus—slightly elevated, pigmented choroidal lesion with overlying drusen.

◆ Choroidal Melanoma

Choroidal melanoma is the most common primary intraocular malignancy. It is characterized by a unilateral, solitary pigmented choroidal mass that shows definite signs of growth over time.

Fundus Features (Figs. 35.2, 35.3, and 35.4)

- ◆ Pigmented (gray-brown) choroidal mass—A small minority of lesions are non-pigmented (amelanotic choroidal melanoma).
  - ◦ >2.5 mm thickness (unlike nevus)
  - ◦ Usually >5 mm diameter
- ◆ Orange pigment (lipofuscin)—visible deposits overlying the lesion
- ◆ Subretinal fluid
- ◆ "Collar-button"–shaped tumor—This configuration results from rupture of Bruch's membrane by an enlarging tumor and is highly typical of choroidal malignant melanoma.
- ◆ Subretinal hemorrhage
- ◆ Vitreous hemorrhage
- ◆ Vitreous pigment

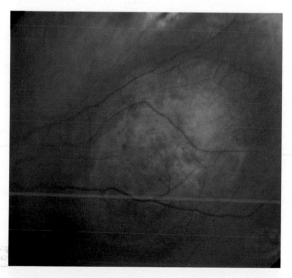

Fig. 35.2 Choroidal malignant melanoma—elevated, pigmented choroidal lesion with overlying orange pigment, suggestive of malignant melanoma.

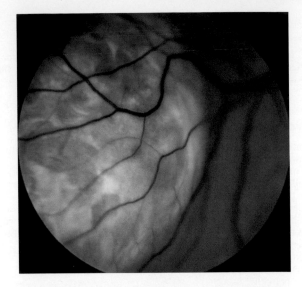

Fig. 35.3 Large malignant melanoma—highly elevated pigmented choroidal lesion with orange pigment deposits characteristic of malignant melanoma. Elevation of the surrounding retina indicates presence of subretinal fluid.

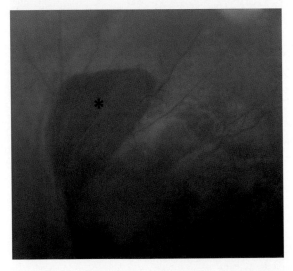

Fig. 35.4 Choroidal malignant melanoma with extension into the subretinal space (*asterisk*). Retinal hemorrhage and subretinal fluid are present.

Other Ophthalmic Features

◆ Blurred vision
◆ Metamorphopsia
◆ Photopsia
◆ Floaters
◆ Relative scotoma
◆ Dilated episcleral vessels ("sentinel" vessels) overlying tumor
◆ Pigment in the anterior chamber
◆ Pigment in trabecular meshwork
◆ Secondary glaucoma

Differential Diagnosis (Fig. 35.5, 35.6, and 35.7; Table 35.1)

◆ Choroidal nevus
◆ Choroidal metastasis
◆ Subretinal or choroidal hemorrhage
◆ Choroidal hemangioma
◆ Melanocytoma
◆ Other pigmented lesions of fundus; e.g., choroidal detachment

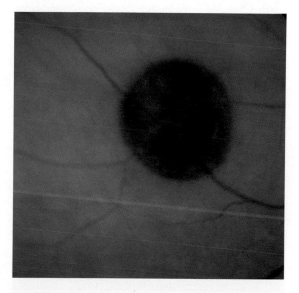

Fig. 35.5 Congenital hypertrophy of the retinal pigment epithelium (CHRPE)—darkly pigmented, flat lesion with well-circumscribed margins and areas of depigmentation. The flat nature of the lesion, its dark coloration, and absence of sub-retinal fluid and orange pigment distinguish this lesion from a malignant melanoma.

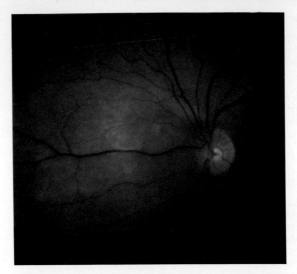

Fig. 35.6 Choroidal hemangioma—dome-shaped, pink-red, elevated choroidal lesion, with a "beaten-brass" appearance of the surface.

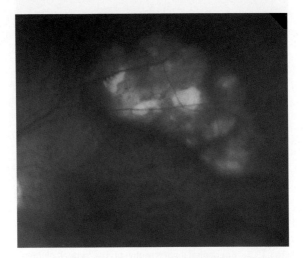

Fig. 35.7 Choroidal osteoma—nonpigmented choroidal mass with overlying areas of retinal pigment epithelium (RPE) and choriocapillary atrophy and variable pigment clumping. B-scan ultrasonography demonstrated a highly echogenic mass with extensive retrobulbar shadowing suggestive of choroidal osteoma.

Table 35.1 Diagnosis of Choroidal Malignant Melanoma

Clinical examination
- ◆ Melanotic (90%) choroidal mass associated with orange pigment and subretinal fluid

B-scan echography
- ◆ Dome-shaped tumor, usually >2.5 mm height; low internal reflectivity. Presence of "collar-button" configuration is almost pathognomonic of choroidal malignant melanoma. Subretinal fluid is often present. B-scan echography is useful in serial measurements of tumor dimensions and for detecting extrascleral extension.

A-scan echography
- ◆ Low to medium reflectivity
- ◆ Accurate measurement of tumor height

Fundus fluorescein angiography
- ◆ Multiple pinpoint spots of early hyperfluorescence
- ◆ Double circulation sign—presence of tumor circulation deep to retinal circulation

Fine-needle aspiration
- ◆ Useful for cases with diagnostic uncertainty

Magnetic resonance imaging (MRI) and computed tomography (CT)
- ◆ Useful for screening for metastasis

◆ Retinoblastoma

Retinoblastoma is a primary tumor of the retina that affects 1/20,000 children. It is responsible for 3% of all childhood malignancies and 30% of primary ocular tumors. Seventy-five percent of cases are unilateral, and 25% are bilateral. Approximately 95% are sporadic, and 15% are germinal mutations. Six percent of cases are familial, with autosomal dominant inheritance. Most bilateral cases have a germinal mutation. Trilateral retinoblastoma is a term used to describe primary tumors of both eyes and the pineal gland.

Fundus Features (Figs. 35.8, 35.9, and 35.10; Table 35.2)

- ◆ Translucent, pinkish-white retinal mass
- ◆ Multiple satellite white retinal lesions
- ◆ Larger tumors have pearly white appearance with superficial and deep vascularization.
- ◆ Obscuration of choroidal blood vessels by tumor
- ◆ Serous retinal detachment
- ◆ Vitreous opacities/seeding
- ◆ Optic disc swelling
  - ○ Papilledema—central nervous system (CNS) involvement
  - ○ Optic nerve infiltration
- ◆ Retinal pigmentary changes
- ◆ Tumor regression (**Fig. 35.11**)
  - ○ Areas of retinal pigment epithelium (RPE) atrophy/hypertrophy (depigmented/pigmented areas)
  - ○ Gray-white tumor with irregular surface
  - ○ "Cottage cheese" or chalky calcified appearance

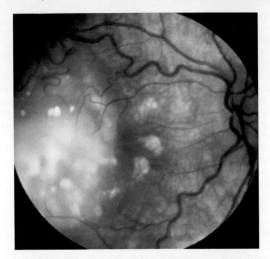

Fig. 35.8   Retinoblastoma—gray-white elevated retinal lesion with areas of calcification. Parts of the tumor appear translucent, characteristic of retinoblastoma.

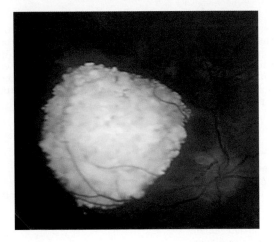

Fig. 35.9   Retinoblastoma—highly elevated chalky-white tumor in a child.

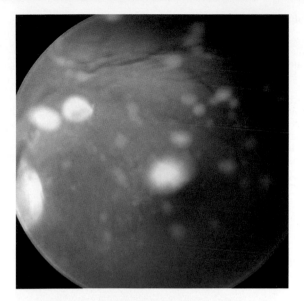

Fig. 35.10 Retinoblastoma—multiple white opacities within the vitreous, indicating vitreous seeding of the retinoblastoma tumor.

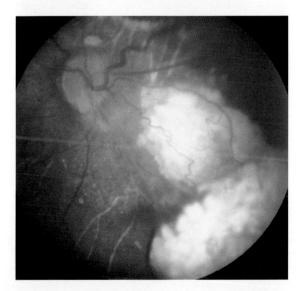

Fig. 35.11 Partially regressed retinoblastoma following chemotherapy—chalky-white, irregular retinal tumor with surrounding area of pigment atrophy and small hemorrhage.

Other Ophthalmic Features

◆ Leukokoria (**Fig. 35.12**)
◆ Infantile strabismus
◆ Spontaneous hyphema
◆ Sterile hypopyon—pseudohypopyon
◆ Uveitis
◆ Heterochromia iridis
◆ Iris neovascularization
◆ Cataract
◆ Secondary glaucoma
◆ Orbital inflammation
◆ Metastasis and extension
  ◦ Optic nerve
  ◦ Orbit—proptosis

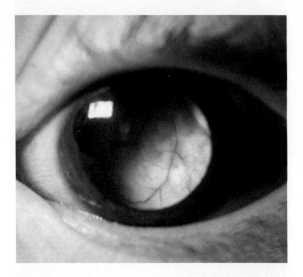

Fig. 35.12   Leukokoria—white pupil reflex in a patient with retinoblastoma. The retinal blood vessels are visible within the pupillary area due to the large tumor elevating the retina.

Systemic Features

◆ Malaise, anorexia, fever, bone pain, weight loss
◆ Other associated primary tumors
  ◦ Osteosarcoma
  ◦ Pinealoma

Table 35.2   Diagnosis of Retinoblastoma

Clinical examination
- ◆ Small tumors are translucent and pinkish-white; larger tumors are pearly white and opaque with superficial and deep vascularization.
- ◆ Multiple or bilateral lesions may be present.
- ◆ Vitreous seeding
- ◆ Systemic signs of malignancy

B-scan echography
- ◆ Single or multiple mass lesions with areas of high reflectivity and acoustic shadowing (calcification)
- ◆ Serous retinal detachment
- ◆ Extension to sclera, optic nerve, and orbit

MRI and CT scan
- ◆ When extraocular or optic nerve spread is suspected

Fine-needle aspiration
- ◆ Usually contraindicated due to risk of tumor tracking

Spinal tap
- ◆ When extraocular or optic nerve spread is suspected

Bone marrow biopsy
- ◆ When extraocular or optic nerve spread is suspected

Genetic studies

Evaluation by pediatric oncologist

◆ Metastasis

Systemic tumors may metastasize to intraocular tissues. Most ocular metastases affect the choroid due to its rich blood supply. Other locations include optic nerve, ciliary body, iris, anterior chamber, conjunctiva, eyelids, extraocular muscles, and orbit. Approximately 25% of patients with uveal or orbital metastasis have no prior history of a primary cancer. The mechanism of metastasis is primarily by hematogenous spread. Diagnostic features are listed in Table 35.3.

Fundus Features (Figs. 35.13, 35.14, and 35.15)

◆ Dome-shaped or flattened, yellow-light brown lesion located deep to the retina. Initially, the lesion may be relatively flat with ill-defined borders. Multiple or bilateral lesions are present in 25% of the cases.
◆ Serous retinal detachment
◆ Secondary RPE changes with patchy areas of hyper- and hypopigmentation ("leopard spotting")
◆ Visual symptoms depend on the location of the tumor within the fundus. Tumors located at the posterior pole are often visually symptomatic.
◆ Retinal pigment epithelial/choroidal folds—particularly if orbital metastasis is causing proptosis
◆ Optic nerve infiltration—pseudopapilledema

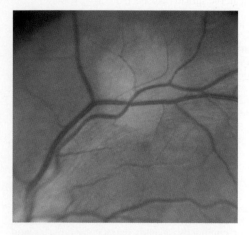

Fig. 35.13 Choroidal metastasis—small, slightly elevated, nonpigmented, yellow choroidal metastasis in a patient with breast carcinoma.

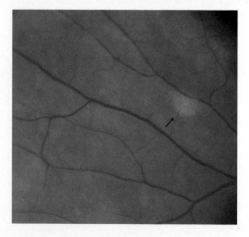

Fig. 35.14 Choroidal metastasis—small, flat, yellow choroidal lesion (*arrow*) in a patient with carcinoid tumor.

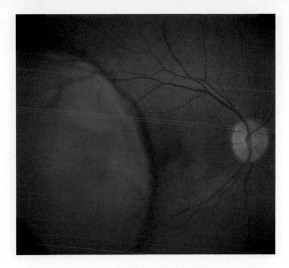

Fig. 35.15 Choroidal metastasis from lung carcinoma—large choroidal mass with surrounding shallow subretinal fluid and macular folds.

Other Ophthalmic Features

◆ Ciliary body tumor
◆ Iris infiltration/mass (**Fig. 35.16**)
◆ Iris neovascularization
◆ Pseudo-iritis
◆ Hyphema
◆ Secondary glaucoma
◆ Conjunctival metastasis
◆ Orbital metastasis—proptosis

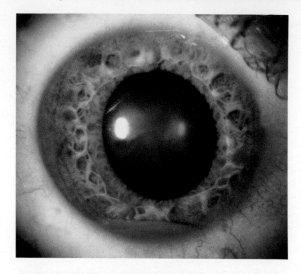

Fig. 35.16 Small metastatic iris lesions (superiorly and inferiorly) from cutaneous malignant melanoma.

Primary Tumors with Choroidal Metastasis

◆ Breast
◆ Lung
◆ Gastrointestinal tract
◆ Prostate
◆ Kidney
◆ Skin
◆ Undetermined primary tumor

Differential Diagnosis of Choroidal Metastasis

◆ Amelanotic melanoma
◆ Amelanotic nevus
◆ Choroidal hemangioma
◆ Choroidal osteoma
◆ Choroidal hemorrhage
◆ Subretinal hemorrhage (e.g., age-related macular degeneration)
◆ Posterior scleritis
◆ Serous retinal detachment
◆ Rhegmatogenous retinal detachment

Table 35.3   Diagnosis of Choroidal Metastasis

Clinical examination
   ◆ Yellow, tan, or cream-colored, sometimes ill-defined choroidal mass
     with subretinal fluid; multiple or bilateral lesions may be present;
     systemic signs of malignancy
B-scan echography
   ◆ Echogenic choroidal mass with ill-defined outline; serous retinal
     detachment is a common finding
A-scan echography
   ◆ Medium to high internal reflectivity
Fine-needle aspiration
   ◆ Useful for cases with diagnostic uncertainty
MRI and CT scan
   ◆ Evaluation of site of primary tumor and other organ metastases

◆ Leukemia

Retinal findings in leukemia result from a variety of pathologic processes, including leukemic infiltration, hyper- and hypocoagulable states, hyperviscosity, immunocompromised state, microembolism, anemia, irradiation, and chemotherapy.

Fundus Features

◆ Retinal hemorrhages (**Fig. 35.17**)
   ◦ Flame-shaped
   ◦ Boat-shaped
   ◦ White-centered (pseudo-Roth spots)
   ◦ Dot and blot hemorrhages
◆ Microaneurysms
◆ Cotton-wool spots
◆ Retinal leukemic infiltrates
◆ Perivascular sheathing/infiltrates (**Fig. 35.18**)
◆ Telangiectasis—usually due to vascular occlusion, radiation retinopathy
◆ Dilated and tortuous retinal vessels
◆ Peripheral retinal neovascularization—typically associated with chronically el-
   evated white blood cell (WBC) count
◆ Retinal vein occlusion
◆ Serous retinal detachment
◆ Pigmentary changes
◆ Vitreous hemorrhage
◆ Vitreous infiltrates
◆ Choroidal infiltrates
◆ Opportunistic infections of choroid, retina, and vitreous
◆ Optic disc
   ◦ Papilledema—elevated intracranial pressure
   ◦ Infiltration
   ◦ Atrophy

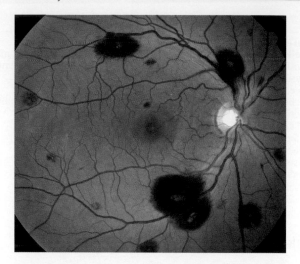

Fig. 35.17 Multiple white-centered retinal hemorrhages in acute leukemia.

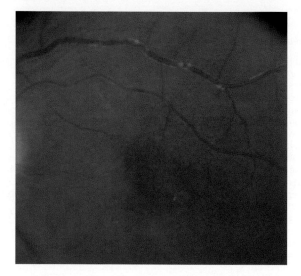

Fig. 35.18 Yellow-white areas of sheathing, indicating perivascular infiltration in a patient with chronic leukemia.

Other Ophthalmic Features

- Conjunctiva
  - Perivascular infiltration
  - Chemosis
  - Subconjunctival hemorrhage
- Cornea
  - Limbal and stromal infiltrates
  - Pannus
- Glaucoma
- Anterior chamber
  - Anterior uveitis
  - Pseudo-hypopyon
  - Heterochromia irides
  - Hyphema
- Orbit and eyelids
  - Infiltration
  - Hemorrhage
  - Orbital and extraocular muscle fibrosis
  - Opportunistic infections
- Cranial nerve palsies
- Complications of treatment
  - Cicatricial lid disease
  - Dry eye
  - Keratoconjunctivitis
  - Keratitis
  - Scleritis
  - Cataract
  - Radiation retinopathy
  - Radiation optic neuropathy
  - Drug-related retinopathy
  - Toxic optic neuropathy

◆ Lymphoma

Intraocular lymphoma is usually the non-Hodgkin variety. Both eyes are affected in 80% of cases. Approximately 20% of cases are limited to the eye; 60% have associated CNS involvement; and 20% have visceral involvement. The most common ocular manifestation is vitreous infiltration masquerading as vitritis.

Fundus Features

◆ Vitreous
  ◦ Lymphoma cell infiltration—diffuse, clumps
  ◦ Vitritis
  ◦ Hemorrhage
◆ Retina
  ◦ Hemorrhages
  ◦ Retinal infiltrates—fuzzy, white, superficial infiltrates
  ◦ Subretinal/sub-RPE infiltrates (**Fig. 35.19**)—multifocal, variable size,
    ◆ Yellow-orange patches, or elevated lesions
    ◆ Mottling at the level of the RPE
  ◦ Perivascular infiltration
  ◦ Retinal vascular occlusion
  ◦ Macular edema
  ◦ Serous retinal detachment
  ◦ RPE atrophy and hyperplasia (**Fig. 35.20**)—late features
◆ Choroid
  ◦ Lymphomatous infiltration
  ◦ Choroidal mass
  ◦ Diffuse or punched-out chorioretinal scars—late feature
◆ Opportunistic infections
◆ Optic disc
  ◦ Papilledema—elevated intracranial pressure
  ◦ Optic nerve infiltration—congested, swollen disc
  ◦ Optic atrophy—late feature

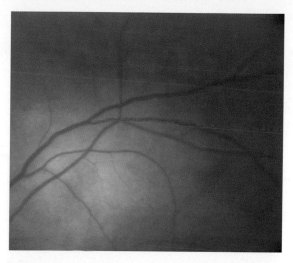

Fig. 35.19 Slightly elevated yellow-orange subretinal lesion with indistinct borders, indicating lymphomatous infiltration in a patient with non-Hodgkin lymphoma.

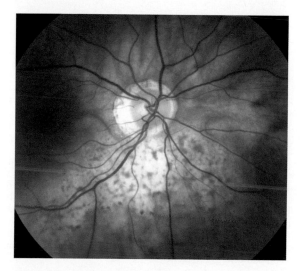

Fig. 35.20 Patchy areas of pigment clumping and atrophy that developed following chemotherapy and regression of subretinal lymphomatous infiltrative lesion. Small patches of residual subretinal infiltrate are present.

Other Ophthalmic Features

◆ Eyelids—lymphomatous infiltration
◆ Conjunctiva—pink subconjunctival mass (salmon-colored lesion) (**Fig. 35.21**)
◆ Cornea—stromal infiltration, keratic precipitates
◆ Anterior uveitis
◆ Iris infiltration/mass
◆ Iris neovascularization
◆ Pseudohypopyon
◆ Lacrimal gland mass
◆ Orbital infiltration—proptosis

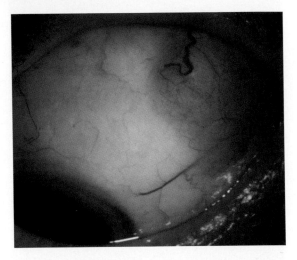

Fig. 35.21   "Salmon-pink" subconjunctival mass characteristic of lymphoma.

◆ Cancer-Associated Retinopathy

Cancer-associated retinopathy (CAR) is a form of retinal degeneration that occurs through a paraneoplastic immunologic mechanism. Symptoms include progressive loss of central or peripheral vision, photopsia, ring scotoma, patchy scotoma, and nyctalopia. Electroretinogram (ERG) is diminished and has negative waveforms. Antirecoverin antibodies may be present.

Melanoma-associated retinopathy (MAR) is a paraneoplastic retinal degeneration that occurs in association with cutaneous malignant melanoma. Autoantibodies to retinal bipolar cells are present.

Fundus Features

◆ Retinal arterial narrowing
◆ Cystoid macular edema
◆ Diffuse or patchy retinal pigment abnormality—a late feature

◆ Radiation Retinopathy

Radiation retinopathy is a delayed-onset, slowly progressive retinal microvasculopathy that resembles diabetic retinopathy. It may occur after external irradiation to the eye or orbit, or after local radioactive plaque therapy. The mean interval to onset is 18 months. Exposure to doses of 30 Gy or more is required. Radiation retinopathy develops in 50% of patients receiving 60 Gy, and in 90% of patients receiving 80 Gy. The total dose and fractionation scheme are important factors influencing the rapidity of onset and severity of radiation retinopathy. Patients present with a variable degree of visual loss.

Fundus Features (Fig. 35.22, 35.23, 35.24, and 35.25)

- ◆ Retinal hemorrhages
  - ◦ Superficial flame-shaped
  - ◦ Dot and blot
  - ◦ Preretinal
- ◆ Microaneurysms
- ◆ Cotton-wool spots
- ◆ Hard Exudates
- ◆ Capillary telangiectasis
- ◆ Retinal vasculitis
- ◆ Capillary nonperfusion—seen on fluorescein angiography
- ◆ Retinal vein occlusion
- ◆ Retinal artery occlusion
- ◆ Perivascular sheathing
- ◆ Retinal neovascularization
- ◆ Macular edema
- ◆ Tractional retinal detachment
- ◆ Choroidal neovascularization resulting in subretinal hemorrhage
- ◆ Vitreous hemorrhage
- ◆ Optic disc swelling—radiation optic neuropathy
- ◆ Optic atrophy

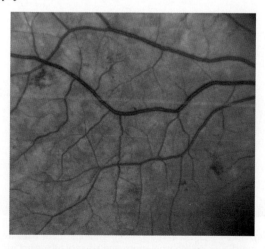

Fig. 35.22 Retinal telangiectasis and retinal hemorrhages in a patient with mild radiation retinopathy.

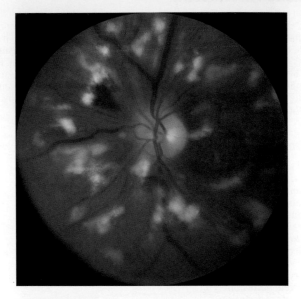

Fig. 35.23 Retinal hemorrhages and extensive cotton-wool spots, indicating microvascular retinopathy following external irradiation.

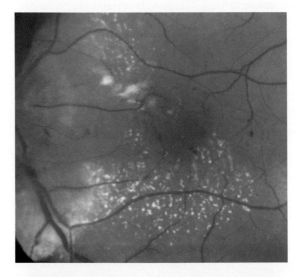

Fig. 35.24 Radiation retinopathy—multiple hard exudates, hemorrhages, cotton-wool spots, and areas of telangiectasis.

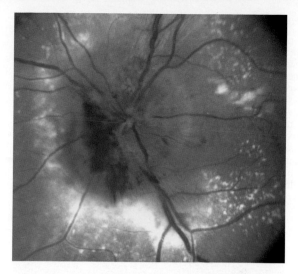

Fig. 35.25 Radiation optic neuropathy—hyperemic and elevated optic disc with surface telangiectasis and hemorrhages, and extensive peripapillary hard exudates, indicating severe radiation optic neuropathy.

Other Ophthalmic Features

◆ Dry-eye syndrome
◆ Cataract
◆ Iris neovascularization
◆ Neovascular glaucoma

◆ Bone Marrow Transplant–Associated Retinopathy

Bone marrow transplant (BMT)-associated retinopathy refers to a group of retinopathies that occur in patients who have undergone BMT. Multiple pathophysiologic mechanisms result in occlusive retinal microvasculopathy, choroidopathy, optic neuropathy, and chorioretinal infections. BMT-associated retinopathy is usually mild and associated with a good prognosis. Treatment is not required in most cases unless serious complications, such as retinal neovascularization or intraocular infections, arise.

Fundus Features

◆ Retinal hemorrhages (**Fig. 35.26**)
◆ Microaneurysms
◆ Cotton-wool spots
◆ Retinal edema and hard exudates
◆ Vascular telangiectasis
◆ Perivascular sheathing
◆ Retinal vascular occlusion
◆ Retinal neovascularization
◆ Tractional retinal detachment
◆ Serous retinal detachment
◆ Infectious chorioretinitis
◆ Endogenous endophthalmitis
◆ Papilledema
◆ Optic atrophy
◆ Vitreous hemorrhage
◆ Vitritis

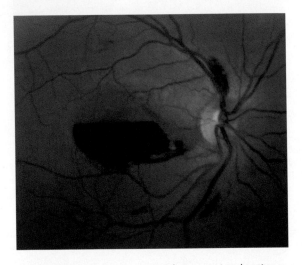

Fig. 35.26 Bone marrow transplant–associated retinopathy—white-centered hemorrhages, retrohyaloid hemorrhage, and cotton-wool spot following allogenic bone marrow transplant for leukemia.

◆ Tamoxifen Retinopathy

Tamoxifen retinopathy is characterized by presence of fine refractile yellow-white deposits within the inner retina layers. Toxicity is rare at the currently used low doses. It may occur at doses >200 mg/day, with a cumulative dose >100 g (see the section on Tamoxifen in Chapter 39).

- Differentiating choroidal nevus from choroidal melanoma.

	Nevus	Malignant Melanoma
Height	≤2 mm	>2.5 mm
Diameter	≤5 mm	>5 mm
Overlying drusen	Often	Occasional
Overlying orange pigment (lipofuscin)	No	Occasional
Subretinal fluid	Occasional	Often
Growth	No	Yes
Laterality	May be bilateral, multiple	Unilateral, solitary lesion
Other		Vitreous pigment
		Vitreous hemorrhage

- Differentiating choroidal melanoma from choroidal metastasis

	Malignant Melanoma	Metastasis
Pigmentation	90% are pigmented (brown/slate-gray)	Yellow/tan/light brown
Shape	Dome-shaped; mushroom-shaped	May be irregular, flat, or occasionally dome-shaped
Laterality	Unilateral	May be bilateral
Number of lesions	Solitary	Solitary or multiple
Subretinal fluid	Yes	Yes
Echography	Low to medium reflectivity	Medium to high reflectivity
Systemic features	Evidence of metastasis (late)	Primary tumor usually detectable

- In children, presence of calcification within an intraocular tumor on B-scan echography or computed tomography (CT) is characteristic of retinoblastoma.

- Risk of developing retinoblastoma

Parent with Parents and siblings not affected	Parent with unilateral retino-blastoma	Sibling with bilateral retino-blastoma	Sibling with unilateral retino-blastoma	bilateral retino-blastoma	>1 Sibling with bilateral retino-blastoma
<0.1%	~10%	~45%	<1%	~5%	~45%

- Differential diagnosis of leukokoria in children:
  - Retinoblastoma
  - Retinopathy of prematurity (ROP)
  - Persistent fetal vasculature (PFV)
  - Retinal astrocytoma
  - Retinal dysplasia
  - Coats disease
  - Toxocariasis
  - Retinal detachment
  - Incontinentia pigmenti resulting in retinal detachment
  - Large retinochoroidal coloboma
  - Familial exudative vitreoretinopathy
  - Congenital cataract
  - Large area of myelinated nerve fibers

- Ocular lymphoma may masquerade as vitritis. Patients with chronic vitritis not responding to anti-inflammatory treatment may require vitreous biopsy to evaluate for ocular lymphoma.

◆ Usher Syndrome (Fig. 36.1)

Usher syndrome is an autosomal recessive disorder characterized by a varying degree of hearing loss, pigmentary retinopathy, and central nervous system abnormalities, including difficulties with balance. Four main subtypes:

Type 1

- Pigmentary retinopathy
- Profound deafness
- Speech impairment
- Vestibular abnormality
- Nonprogressive ataxia
- Onset in childhood
- Legally blind by fourth decade of life

Type 2

- Pigmentary retinopathy
- Moderate hearing loss—nonprogressive
- Mild or no speech impairment
- Vestibular function intact
- Onset in second decade of life
- Preservation of vision until sixth decade of life

Type 3 (Hallgren Syndrome)

- Pigmentary retinopathy
- Profound deafness
- Ataxia—mild
- Cataract
- Mental retardation—variable
- Schizophrenia

Type 4

- Pigmentary retinopathy
- Profound deafness
- Ataxia
- Cataract
- Mental retardation—marked

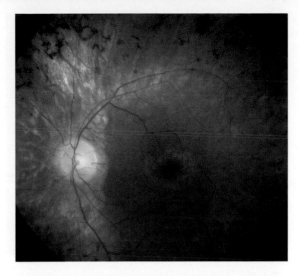

Fig. 36.1 Usher syndrome—bone spicule pigmentary retinopathy, attenuated retinal vessels, and mild waxy pallor of the optic disc in a patient with retinitis pigmentosa and Usher syndrome. Choroidal vessels are visible in the areas with diffuse retinal pigment epithelial atrophy.

Differential Diagnosis of Pigmentary Retinopathy Associated with Deafness

- Usher syndrome
- Congenital rubella
- Congenital syphilis
- Refsum's disease
- Kearns-Sayre syndrome (**Fig. 36.2**)
- Hurler syndrome
- Alström syndrome
- Cockayne syndrome
- Friedreich ataxia
- Flynn-Aird syndrome
- Osteopetrosis

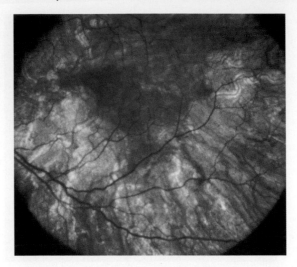

Fig. 36.2   Diffuse retinal pigment epithelial atrophy, making the choroidal vessels visible in a patient with Kearns-Sayre syndrome.

◆ Cogan Syndrome

Cogan syndrome affects young adults and is characterized by interstitial keratitis, neurosensory hearing loss, vestibular dysfunction, and systemic vasculitis (including aortitis).

Ophthalmic Features

- ◆ Papillitis
- ◆ Serous retinal detachment
- ◆ Retinal vasculitis
- ◆ Uveitis
- ◆ Scleritis
- ◆ Episcleritis
- ◆ Orbital pseudotumor
- ◆ Interstitial keratitis—most common ocular feature

◆ Shaken Baby Syndrome/Child Abuse

Shaken baby syndrome is the term used to describe injuries from child abuse that were sustained as a result of episodes of sudden acceleration/deceleration (e.g., shaking of the child). Although child abuse can occur at any age, shaken baby syndrome typically occurs in children under 2 years of age.

Fundus Features (Figs. 37.1, 37.2, and 37.3)

- ◆ Intraretinal folds—circumferential with the optic disc or macula. This is an important sign that indicates shearing forces of sudden acceleration/deceleration. Intraretinal folds are highly suggestive of shaken baby syndrome.
- ◆ Superficial flame-shaped hemorrhages
- ◆ Patchy intraretinal hemorrhages
- ◆ Preretinal, retrohyaloid hemorrhages
- ◆ Subretinal hemorrhages
- ◆ Vitreous hemorrhage
- ◆ Retinoschisis
- ◆ Retinal detachment
- ◆ Pigmentary changes
- ◆ Chorioretinal scars
- ◆ Optic nerve
  - ◦ Hemorrhages
  - ◦ Papilledema
  - ◦ Optic atrophy

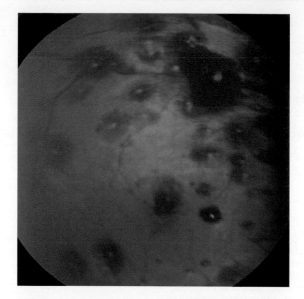

Fig. 37.1 Multiple white-centered and flame-shaped hemorrhages in a patient with shaken baby syndrome.

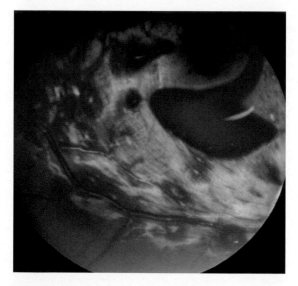

Fig. 37.2 Shaken baby syndrome—retrohyaloid and white-centered hemorrhages, and whitening of the retina, indicating diffuse retinal edema.

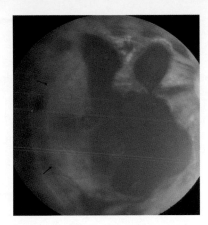

Fig. 37.3 Shaken baby syndrome. Retinal folds (*arrows*), circumferential with the fovea, are highly suggestive of shaken baby syndrome. Retrohyaloid and flame-shaped hemorrhages are also present.

Other Ophthalmic Features of Child Abuse

◆ Signs of periorbital trauma
◆ Proptosis
◆ Orbital fractures
◆ Subconjunctival/conjunctival hemorrhage
◆ Conjunctival/corneal laceration.
◆ Conjunctival/corneal chemical or thermal injuries
◆ Corneal vascularization, opacities
◆ Hyphema
◆ Iritis
◆ Irregular pupil, iridodialysis, angle recession
◆ Lens dislocation and cataract
◆ Strabismus—paralytic, nonparalytic
◆ Glaucoma
◆ Open globe injury
◆ Visual abnormalities
  ◦ Loss of vision—due to ocular, optic nerve, or occipital injuries
  ◦ Amblyopia
  ◦ Atypical visual field defects

Systemic Features

◆ General
  ◦ Irritable, anxious child
  ◦ Delayed medical care
  ◦ Failure to thrive
  ◦ Inconsistent medical history
  ◦ History of multiple episodes of trauma
◆ Musculoskeletal
  ◦ Age-inappropriate multiple fractures at varying stages of healing
  ◦ Spiral fractures of long bones
  ◦ Rib fractures
  ◦ Metaphyseal injury/epiphyseal dislocation
  ◦ Periosteal hemorrhages
  ◦ Skull fractures

- Skin
  - Bruises, burns, lacerations
    - Age-inappropriate injury
    - Multiple, varying stages of healing
    - Atypical location
- Central nervous system
  - Hemorrhage—subdural, subarachnoid, intracerebral, and intraventricular
  - Cerebral edema
  - Contusion injury of frontal and occipital lobes
  - Seizure
  - Cerebral atrophy
  - Developmental delay

◆ Retinopathy of Prematurity

Retinopathy of prematurity (ROP) is a form of retinal vasculopathy that occurs in prematurely born infants as a result of immature retinal vasculature at birth.

Risk Factors for Development of Retinopathy of Prematurity

- Short gestational age—especially <32 weeks
- Low birth weight—<1500 g, especially <1250 g
- Prolonged use of high concentrations of oxygen
- Episodes of hypoxemia, hypercarbia
- Multisystem disease
- Severe, multiple episodes of systemic acidosis
- Septicemia
- Paraventricular, white matter hemorrhages

Fundus Features

- Avascular peripheral retina
- Demarcation line
- Demarcation ridge (**Fig. 37.4**)
- Retinal neovascularization (**Fig. 37.5**)
- Retinal hemorrhage
- Retinal detachment (**Fig. 37.6**)
- Vitreous hemorrhage
- Cicatricial retinopathy—late complication
  - Peripheral vascular anastomoses (**Fig. 37.7**)
  - Retinal folds (**Fig. 37.8**)
  - Vascular dragging
    - "Dragging" of macula (**Fig. 37.9**)
    - "Dragging" of optic disc
  - Tractional retinal detachment
  - Rhegmatogenous retinal detachment
  - Chorioretinal scars
  - Retrolental mass (**Fig. 37.10**)

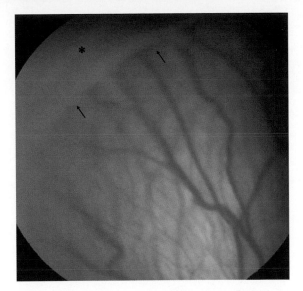

Fig. 37.4 Retinopathy of prematurity, stage 2. An elevated ridge (*arrows*) separates the peripheral avascular retina (*asterisk*) from the vascularized retina posterior to the ridge.

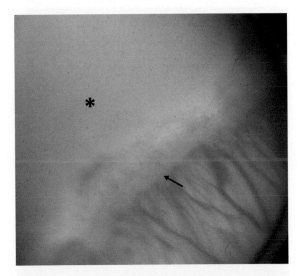

Fig. 37.5 Retinopathy of prematurity, stage 3. An elevated ridge with neovascularization and hemorrhage is present (*arrow*). The retina anterior to this ridge is totally avascular (*asterisk*).

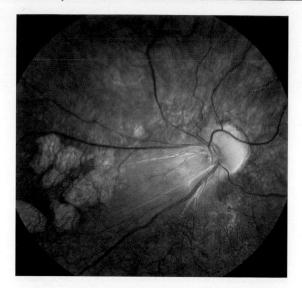

Fig. 37.6 Retinopathy of prematurity (ROP)—tractional retinal detachment and extensive "dragging" of the macula.

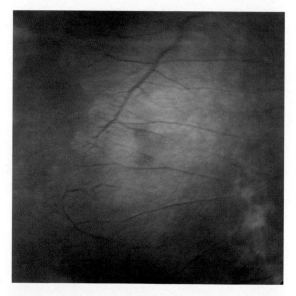

Fig. 37.7 Avascular peripheral retina with abrupt termination of vessels and arteriovenous anastomoses in a 13-year-old patient with history of retinopathy of prematurity.

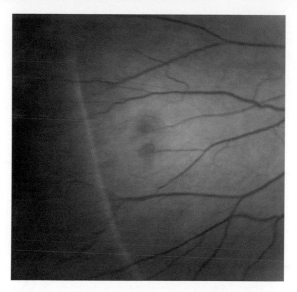

Fig. 37.8 Peripheral retinal fold in a patient with history of retinopathy of prematurity. The peripheral retina is fully vascularized.

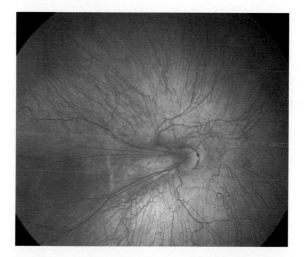

Fig. 37.9 Temporal "dragging" of the macular and optic disc blood vessels in a patient with history of retinopathy of prematurity.

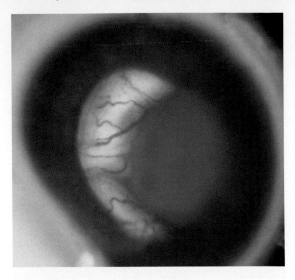

Fig. 37.10   Leukokoria due to retinopathy of prematurity, stage 5—extensively detached retina is visible through the pupil.

Other Ophthalmic Features of Retinopathy of Prematurity

◆ Myopia
◆ Astigmatism
◆ Anisometropia
◆ Amblyopia
◆ Strabismus and pseudostrabismus
◆ Glaucoma
◆ Cataract
◆ Neuro-ophthalmologic
  ◦ Visual field defects
  ◦ Nystagmus
  ◦ Optic atrophy

Classification of Retinopathy of Prematurity

Classification of ROP is based on the location, extent, and stage of the disease and other signs of vascular incompetence (i.e., "plus" disease).

Location

◆ Zone I: a circle with a radius of 5 disc diameters (DD) centered on the optic disc
◆ Zone II: a circle extending from the circle of zone I to the nasal ora serrata
◆ Zone III: the remaining temporal peripheral retina

Extent

Extent refers to the number of clock hours involved, which may be contiguous or cumulative.

Stage

◆ Stage 1: demarcation line, which is a flat white line within the plane of the retina that separates the central (posterior) vascularized retina from the peripheral (anterior) nonvascularized retina
◆ Stage 2: ridge, which is a pink-white demarcation line that appears elevated and has height, width, and volume
◆ Stage 3: extraretinal fibrovascular proliferation at the ridge (**Fig. 37.11**)
◆ Stage 4: subtotal retinal detachment
    A. Extrafoveal (**Fig. 37.12**)
    B. Involving the fovea (**Fig. 37.13**)
◆ Stage 5: total retinal detachment

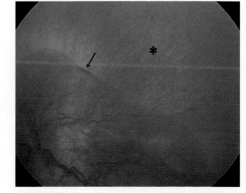

Fig. 37.11 Retinopathy of prematurity, stage 3, zone I. Neovascularization (*arrow*) is present at the ridge in this patient with zone I disease. Dilated and tortuous retinal vessels indicate "plus" disease. Extensive area of avascular retina (*asterisk*) is present peripheral to the ridge.

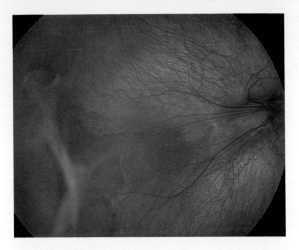

Fig. 37.12 Retinopathy of prematurity, stage 4A—temporal tractional retinal detachment extending centrally, but not involving the macula.

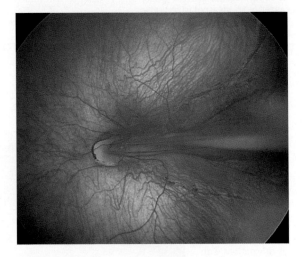

Fig. 37.13 Retinopathy of prematurity, stage 4B—retinal detachment extending centrally to involve the macula.

"Plus" Disease (Fig. 37.14)

"Plus" disease is defined by the presence of dilated and tortuous retinal vessels. It indicates vascular incompetence and a high risk for progression of retinopathy. Neovascularization in zone I with "plus" disease suggests a high risk for rapidly progressive disease ("rush" disease).

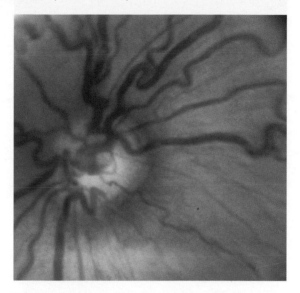

Fig. 37.14 Retinopathy of prematurity—dilated and tortuous retinal vessels, indicating the presence of "plus" disease.

Screening for Retinopathy of Prematurity

Infants weighing less than 1500 g or with less than 36 weeks' gestation should have screening for retinopathy of prematurity.

◆ Initial fundus examination
  ° 4 to 6 weeks after birth
◆ Subsequent fundus examination and management
  ° Completely vascularized retina—comprehensive eye examination at 3 months post-term
  ° Stages 1 to 2, zone III—examination every 2 to 3 weeks until the retina is fully vascularized
  ° Stages 1 to 2, zone II—examination every 2 weeks until the retina is fully vascularized
  ° Stages 1 to 2, zone I—examination every week until the retina is fully vascularized
  ° Stage 3, subthreshold ROP—examination every week until the retina is fully vascularized
  ° Stage 3, threshold ROP—retinal laser photocoagulation to the area of avascular retina (**Fig. 37.15**)
  ° Stage 4 ROP—scleral buckle procedure or vitrectomy
  ° Stage 5 ROP—vitrectomy

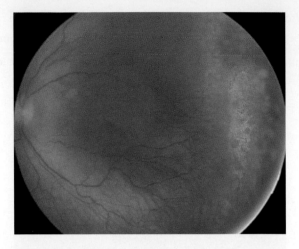

Fig. 37.15   Stage 3 retinopathy of prematurity 2 weeks after treatment with retinal laser photocoagulation. Laser photocoagulation scars are present peripheral to the ridge.

◆ Congenital and Neonatal Infections

Congenital Toxoplasmosis

- ◆ Chorioretinal scars—pigmented scars in the macula or the periphery (**Fig. 37.16**)
- ◆ Vitreous opacities
- ◆ Cataract
- ◆ Microphthalmia
- ◆ Glaucoma
- ◆ Recurrent retinochoroiditis in later life

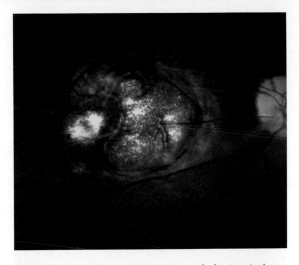

Fig. 37.16 Large, excavated, pigmented chorioretinal scar involving the central macular region of a patient with history of congenital toxoplasmosis. The term macular coloboma is often used to describe this type of excavated scar in congenital toxoplasmosis.

Rubella

Fundus Features

◆ "Salt-and-pepper" retinopathy. A mild form of pigmentary retinopathy with little visual impairment (**Figs. 37.17**). The retinal vasculature and optic disc usually appear normal. Electroretinogram is usually within normal limits. Vision may become impaired by development of choroidal neovascularization in adulthood.
◆ Choroidal neovascularization in adulthood
◆ Absent foveal reflex
◆ Retinal detachment—rare

Other Ophthalmic Features

◆ Congenital cataract
◆ Corneal opacity
◆ Iris hypoplasia
◆ Uveitis
◆ Congenital glaucoma
◆ Optic nerve
  ◦ Optic neuritis
  ◦ Optic atrophy
  ◦ Optic nerve hypoplasia
◆ Refractive errors
◆ Microphthalmia

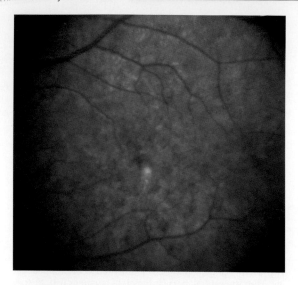

Fig. 37.17 "Salt-and-pepper" pigmentary retinopathy in a 32-year-old patient with congenital rubella. There is no attenuation of the retinal vasculature. The vision was near normal. Electrophysiologic tests were within the normal range.

Systemic Features

- Sensorineural hearing loss
- Psychomotor retardation
- Mental retardation
- Congenital heart disease
  - Patent ductus arteriosus
  - Pulmonary artery stenosis
  - Ventricular and atrial septal defect
  - Aortic coarctation
- Thyroid disease
- Dental and maxillofacial abnormalities
- Hepatosplenomegaly
- Genitourinary abnormalities
- Interstitial pneumonitis
- Growth retardation

Cytomegalovirus

Fundus Features

◆ Active
  ° Retinitis/choroiditis—less severe than acquired cytomegalovirus (CMV) retinitis
  ° Vitritis
  ° Optic neuritis
◆ Late
  ° Chorioretinal scars
  ° Pigmented retinopathy
  ° Optic atrophy
  ° Retinal detachment

Other Ophthalmic Features

◆ Microphthalmia
◆ Optic nerve hypoplasia
◆ Coloboma
◆ Cataract
◆ Glaucoma

Herpes Simplex: Congenital (Intrauterine Infection)

Fundus Features

◆ "Salt-and-pepper" retinopathy
◆ Diffuse or patchy chorioretinal scars
◆ Optic atrophy
◆ Narrowing of retinal vessels

Systemic Features

◆ Central nervous system (CNS)—encephalitis, microcephaly, psychomotor retardation
◆ Skin pigmentation, fibrosis, soft nails
◆ Congenital heart disease

Herpes Simplex: Neonatal (Acquired Infection at Birth)

Fundus Features

◆ Retinitis—creamy-yellow patchy areas of retinitis
◆ Chorioretinitis
◆ Vitritis—hazy vitreous with inflammatory cells
◆ Retinal hemorrhages
◆ Retinal vasculitis
◆ Retinal vascular occlusion
◆ Retinal neovascularization
◆ Retinal detachment
◆ Optic neuritis
◆ Optic atrophy
◆ Narrowing of retinal vessels

Systemic Features

◆ CNS—encephalitis, temporal lobe seizures, psychomotor retardation
◆ Rhinitis
◆ Hepatitis
◆ Hepatosplenomegaly
◆ Glomerulonephritis
◆ Enteritis
◆ Esophagitis

Congenital (Intrauterine) Herpes Zoster

Fundus Features

◆ Pigmentary retinopathy
◆ Chorioretinal scars
◆ Optic atrophy

Other Ocular Features

◆ Cataracts
◆ Microphthalmia

Systemic Features

◆ CNS—cerebral atrophy, microcephaly, psychomotor retardation, seizures
◆ Skin scarring
◆ Low birth weight

Congenital Syphilis

Early

◆ Chorioretinitis
◆ Keratoconjunctivitis

Late

◆ Chorioretinal scars
◆ "Salt-and-pepper" retinopathy
◆ Attenuated retinal vasculature
◆ Optic atrophy
◆ Uveitis
◆ Interstitial keratitis
◆ Hutchinson triad
  ○ Interstitial keratitis
  ○ Neurosensory hearing loss
  ○ Hutchinson teeth—peg-shaped teeth with a crescent-shaped notch

Pearls

- Findings suggestive of shaken baby syndrome
  - Intraretinal folds
  - Extensive retinal hemorrhages in the absence of apparent head, periorbital, or ocular injuries
  - Retinal hemorrhages and history of repetitive, multiorgan injuries

- In premature, low birth weight infants, progression of ROP correlates with the infant's general state of health. Premature infants with severe hypoxia, septicemia, and other intercurrent disease need to be monitored closely for progression of ROP.

- In addition to ROP and its sequelae, prematurely born infants are susceptible to development of other ophthalmic abnormalities, such as refractive errors, amblyopia, strabismus, glaucoma, and retinal detachment. They require regular ophthalmological evaluations throughout life.

Fundus Features

- ◆ Hypertensive retinopathy (eclampsia/preeclampsia)
  - ◦ Focal/diffuse narrowing of retinal arterioles
  - ◦ Flame-shaped, dot-and-blot hemorrhages
  - ◦ Microaneurysms
  - ◦ Cotton-wool spots
  - ◦ Retinal edema
  - ◦ Hard exudates
  - ◦ Serous retinal detachment
  - ◦ Choroidal infarcts
  - ◦ Choroidal scars—late feature
  - ◦ Optic disc edema
- ◆ Purtscher-like retinopathy (**Fig. 38.1**)
  - ◦ Blurred vision

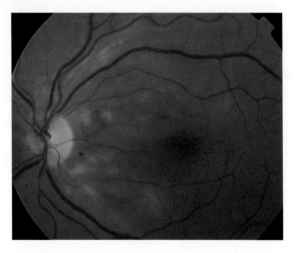

Fig. 38.1 Purtscher-like retinopathy following prolonged labor in a 27-year-old woman. Multiple cotton-wool spots and minor hemorrhages are present.

- ◆ Cotton-wool spots, especially in the peripapillary region
- ◆ Superficial flame-shaped retinal hemorrhages
- ◆ Good visual recovery with resolution of retinopathy
- ◆ Associated with:
  - ◦ Amniotic fluid embolism
  - ◦ Disseminated intravascular coagulopathy (DIC)
  - ◦ Blood/platelet transfusion

- ◆ Valsalva retinopathy
  - ◦ Retinal, subretinal, retrohyaloid, and vitreous hemorrhages
- ◆ Central serous chorioretinopathy
- ◆ Serous/exudative retinal detachment (**Fig. 38.2**)
  - ◦ Preeclampsia/eclampsia
  - ◦ Postpartum
- ◆ Progression of diabetic retinopathy

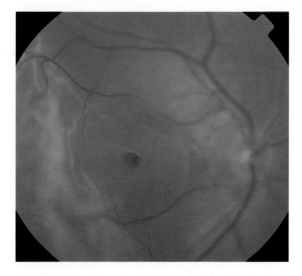

Fig. 38.2 Extensive serous retinal detachment occurring soon after labor in a patient with preeclampsia. The visual acuity was 20/400. The retinal detachment resolved spontaneously within 6 weeks, and visual acuity improved to 20/25.

Other Ophthalmic Features

- ◆ Blurring of vision—mild
- ◆ Refractive changes
- ◆ Reduced corneal sensation
- ◆ Change in corneal thickness
- ◆ Contact lens intolerance
- ◆ Periorbital/eyelid swelling
- ◆ Neuro-ophthalmologic
  - ◦ Horner syndrome—after spinal anesthesia
  - ◦ Migraine—worsened by pregnancy
  - ◦ Pituitary enlargement/apoplexy
  - ◦ Occipital blindness—due to occipital cortex infarction
  - ◦ Enlargement of meningioma
  - ◦ Intracranial venous/sinus thrombosis
  - ◦ Idiopathic intracranial hypertension (pseudotumor cerebri)

Pearls

- Rapid progression of diabetic retinopathy may occur during pregnancy. Patients with diabetic retinopathy who become pregnant require close monitoring of the retinopathy.

39 Drug-Related Retinopathy

◆ Hydroxychloroquine (Plaquenil)/Chloroquine

Retinal toxicity occurs more frequently with chloroquine than hydroxychloroquine. Chloroquine toxicity is more likely to occur if the total cumulative dose is >300 g, and the daily dose is >250 mg. For hydroxychloroquine, daily doses of >400 mg have the potential to cause toxicity, although severe damage is rare. Pigmentary maculopathy of variable severity is present in 30% of patients who are on very high cumulative doses of hydroxychloroquine. Macular damage may occur before there are ophthalmoscopic signs. Visual symptoms in the early stages may be reversed by cessation of the drug. In advanced stages, toxic effects may progress despite discontinuation of medication.

Fundus Features

- Mild pigment stippling in the macular region
- "Bull's-eye" maculopathy (**Figs. 39.1 and 39.2**)—hypopigmented and hyperpigmented rings of retinal pigment epithelium (RPE) atrophy and hypertrophy surrounding the foveal region. "Bull's-eye" maculopathy represents advanced toxicity.
- Peripheral pigmentary abnormalities
- Fundus fluorescein angiography demonstrates rings of hyper- and hypofluorescence corresponding to the "bull's eye" maculopathy.

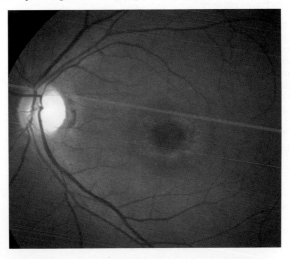

Fig. 39.1 Annular area of retinal pigmentary disturbance centered on the fovea in a patient on long-term treatment with hydroxychloroquine.

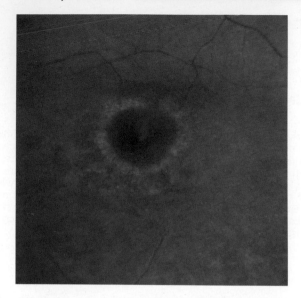

Fig. 39.2 "Bull's-eye" maculopathy—concentric hyperpigmented and hypopigmented rings of retinal pigment epithelial hypertrophy and atrophy in a patient on long-term hydroxychloroquine therapy.

Other Ophthalmic Features

◆ Symptoms
  ○ Asymptomatic in early stages
  ○ Blurred vision
  ○ Abnormal color vision
  ○ Relative scotomas
◆ Abnormal central visual field—especially red color field
◆ Corneal deposits
◆ Abnormal electroretinogram

Risk Factors for Development of Retinal Toxicity

◆ High daily dose
◆ High total (cumulative) dose
◆ Prolonged treatment
◆ Advanced age
◆ Low body weight
◆ Preexisting macular disease

◆ Phenothiazines

Phenothiazines are concentrated in uveal tissue and RPE by binding to melanin granules. In high concentrations they can interfere with RPE function.

Chlorpromazine (Thorazine)

- ◆ Visually asymptomatic in early stages
- ◆ Pigmentary retinopathy—occurs with high dose (>2400 mg/day for over 1 year)
- ◆ Abnormal pigmentation
  - ◦ Eyelids
  - ◦ Conjunctiva
  - ◦ Cornea
  - ◦ Lens

◆ Thioridazine (Mellaril)

Thioridazine retinal toxicity typically occurs after prolonged therapy. High-dose therapy (>800 mg/day) may result in toxicity within weeks of starting medication. Once established, toxicity may progress despite discontinuation of the drug.

Fundus Features

- ◆ Mild pigment stippling—early stages
- ◆ Severe pigmentary retinopathy—late stages
- ◆ Patchy areas of RPE and choriocapillary atrophy—late stages

Other Ophthalmic Features

- ◆ Blurred vision
- ◆ Altered color vision
- ◆ Night blindness
- ◆ Visual field loss
- ◆ Pigment deposits in cornea and anterior lens

◆ Tamoxifen

Tamoxifen is an antiestrogen agent used in treatment of breast cancer. Tamoxifen retinopathy is rare at the currently used low doses of 10 to 20 mg/day. Toxicity may occur at doses greater than 200 mg/day, and with cumulative doses over 100 g. Symptoms improve after discontinuation of the drug.

Fundus Features (Figs. 39.3 and 39.4)

◆ Fine refractile yellow-white deposits in superficial perifoveal retina
◆ Cystoid macular edema
◆ Subtle punctate macular pigmentary changes
◆ RPE and choriocapillary atrophy—late stages of severe cases

Other Ophthalmic Features

◆ Blurred vision—usually mild
◆ Subtle color vision abnormalities
◆ Fine corneal subepithelial opacities

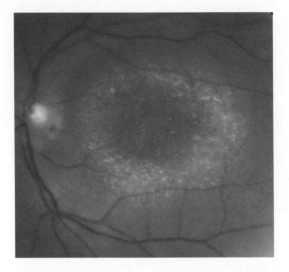

Fig. 39.3 Tamoxifen retinopathy—multiple fine yellow-white deposits within the superficial retina in a patient on high-dose therapy for breast carcinoma.

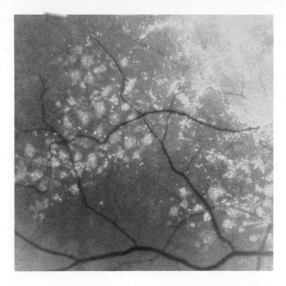

Fig. 39.4 Tamoxifen retinopathy—extensive, yellow-white, refractile intraretinal deposits in tamoxifen toxicity.

◆ Canthaxanthine

Canthaxanthine is a carotenoid used to simulate tanning of the skin. High doses of canthaxanthine can cause a crystalline maculopathy. The condition is usually asymptomatic and improves on stopping the medication.

Fundus Features

- ◆ "Gold dust" maculopathy—doughnut-shaped pattern of fine crystals in superficial retina
- ◆ Pigmentary maculopathy—severe cases

Other Ophthalmic Features

- ◆ Corneal crystalline deposits

◆ Interferon

Interferon α is used in treatment of chronic hepatitis C, melanoma, and Kaposi sarcoma, and is included in many chemotherapy protocols. Interferon-associated retinopathy is usually asymptomatic and self-limiting, with spontaneous improvement after cessation of the drug. Occasionally, vision may become adversely affected. Interferon retinopathy typically occurs within the first 4 to 6 weeks of starting therapy. It is seen more frequently in diabetic and hypertensive patients.

Fundus Features

- Cotton wool spots (**Fig. 39.5**)
- Retinal hemorrhages
- Macular edema
- Optic disc edema
- Arterial and venous occlusion

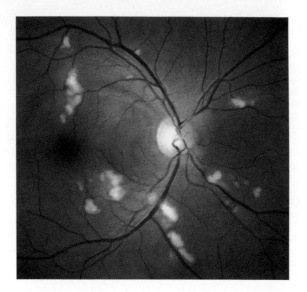

Fig. 39.5 Interferon retinopathy—multiple cotton-wool spots in a patient on interferon α therapy. The patient was asymptomatic.

◆ Isotretinoin (Accutane)

Isotretinoin (Accutane) is used for treatment of acne. Prolonged use may result in night vision difficulties with abnormal dark-adaptation. The electroretinography (ERG) response becomes abnormal. The condition improves after cessation of drug.

◆ Methoxyflurane Anesthesia

Methoxyflurane can cause a form of crystalline retinopathy as a result of deposition of oxalate crystals (secondary oxalosis). Typically, the vision is normal. Fine yellow-white crystal deposits are present at the macula and the mid-periphery, often in a paravascular distribution.

◆ Talc

Talc or cornstarch fillers in crushed tablets taken intravenously by drug abusers can cause a microembolic retinopathy with crystal deposition. In severe cases, talc retinopathy may resemble sickle cell retinopathy with peripheral retinal vascular proliferation.

Fundus Features

◆ White-yellow crystalline deposits (**Fig. 39.6**)
◆ Areas of capillary closure
◆ Retinal hemorrhages, cotton-wool spots
◆ Peripheral retinal neovascularization
◆ Vitreous hemorrhage, tractional retinal detachment

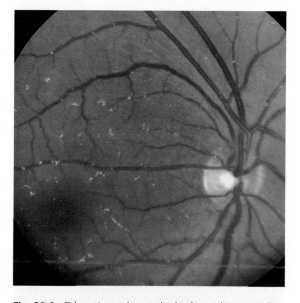

Fig. 39.6   Talc retinopathy—multiple, fine, white crystalline deposits, predominantly concentrated in the proximity of the larger retinal vessels, in a patient with history of intravenous drug abuse.

◆ Other Drug-Related Retinal and Optic Nerve Toxicities

Cardiac Glycosides (Digitalis)

High doses of digoxin result in cone dysfunction, causing blurred vision, pericentral scotoma, and xanthopsia (yellow vision). There is no visible retinopathy. The effects are reversed with cessation of the drug.

Sildenafil (Viagra)

High doses of sildenafil cause transient "blue" tinting of vision. Sildenafil may possibly cause optic neuropathy.

2',3'-Dideoxyinosine

2',3'-Dideoxyinosine (DDI) is an antiviral agent used in the treatment of AIDS. It may cause a mid-peripheral pigmentary retinopathy that improves after discontinuation of medication.
- ◆ Blurred vision
- ◆ Night vision difficulty
- ◆ Mid-peripheral pigmentary retinopathy
- ◆ Abnormal ERG and electro-oculography (EOG)

Carbamazepine (Tegretol)

Very high cumulative doses of carbamazepine may cause bread crumb–like flecks in deep retina, RPE abnormalities, blurred vision, and visual field defects (**Fig. 39.7**).

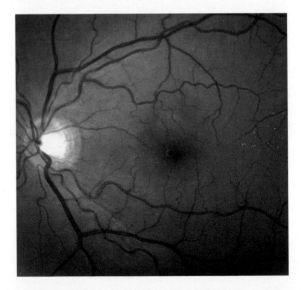

Fig. 39.7 Multiple, fine, yellow subretinal deposits in a patient on long-term carbamazepine.

Cisplatin, Carmustine

Cisplatin and carmustine (BCNU) are chemotherapeutic agents used in the treatment of various malignancies. They can cause retinopathy and optic neuropathy.
- Pigmentary maculopathy
- Macular edema
- Cotton-wool spots
- Retinal hemorrhages
- Vascular occlusion
- Vasculitis
- Optic neuropathy

Deferoxamine

Deferoxamine is used for treatment of iron overload in patients who receive multiple blood transfusions. Deferoxamine causes diffuse pigmentary retinopathy, macular edema, visual loss, nyctalopia, visual field loss, and abnormal ERG and EOG. Return of visual function occurs with cessation of medication.

Nicotinic Acid

High-dose nicotinic acid has been used for treatment of hyperlipidemia. It can cause blurred vision, paracentral scotoma, and cystoid macular edema. Fluorescein angiography fails to demonstrate vascular leakage in the area of the cystoid edema.

Nitrofurantoin

Nitrofurantoin is associated with crystalline retinopathy and optic neuropathy.

Rifabutin

Rifabutin is associated with anterior and posterior uveitis. Uveitis resolves on stopping the medication.

Cidofovir

Cidofovir may cause uveitis and ocular hypotony.

Pearls

- Because early stages of hydroxychloroquine maculopathy may be asymptomatic, regular, routine screening is prudent. Screening methods consist of eye examinations every 6 months, including visual acuity, color vision, Amsler grid, fundus examination, static perimetry, and macular red color visual field testing. In cases suspected of toxicity, multifocal ERG and EOG studies may help with establishing the diagnosis.

- Color vision testing (e.g., Ishihara color plates) is useful in early detection of drug-related optic neuropathy. A relative afferent pupillary defect may not be clinically apparent due to the bilateral and often symmetrical nature of the condition.

- Differential diagnosis of "bull's-eye" maculopathy
  - Chloroquine/hydroxychloroquine maculopathy
  - Cone dystrophy
  - Stargardt disease
  - Age-related macular degeneration
  - Tamoxifen retinopathy
  - Canthaxanthine maculopathy
  - Phototoxicity
  - Benign concentric annular macular dystrophy
  - Adult vitelliform dystrophy
  - Batten disease
  - Olivopontocerebellar degeneration
  - Spielmeyer-Vogt syndrome

- Drugs associated with pigmentary retinopathy
  - Chloroquine/hydroxychloroquine (Plaquenil)
  - Phenothiazines—thioridazine (Mellaril), chlorpromazine (Thorazine)
  - Carbamazepine (Tegretol)
  - Ethambutol
  - Indomethacin
  - Penicillamine
  - Deferoxamine
  - Chemotherapeutic agents—cisplatin, carmustine
  - 2',3'-dideoxyinosine (DDI)

- Drugs associated with optic neuropathy
  - Ethambutol
  - Isoniazid
  - Amiodarone
  - Sildenafil (Viagra)
  - Chloramphenicol
  - Sulfonamides
  - Cisplatin, carmustine
  - Vincristine
  - Penicillamine
  - Hydroxyquinolines
  - Barbiturates

◆ Age-Related Macular Degeneration

Age-related macular degeneration (AMD) is the most common cause of severe visual loss in developed countries. There are two main forms:

◆ Nonexudative AMD—"dry" AMD
◆ Exudative AMD—"wet" AMD

Nonexudative AMD may progress to exudative AMD, which in turn may progress to disciform scarring (end-stage AMD).

Nonexudative ("Dry")

Nonexudative ("dry") AMD is a bilateral condition affecting individuals older than 50 years of age. Most individuals are asymptomatic at the time of diagnosis. Some patients experience gradual loss of visual acuity, mild distortion of central vision, or small central or paracentral scotomas.

Fundus Features

◆ Drusen (**Figs. 40.1 and 40.2**)—multiple, typically nonrefractile focal, yellow or cream-colored subretinal deposits. Old calcified drusen may appear refractile. Drusen occur primarily at the macular region, but may also occur in the periphery.
◆ Pigment clumping—irregular clumps of brown pigment, often interspersed with drusen, in the central macular region
◆ Focal, patchy areas of retinal pigment epithelial (RPE) atrophy—appear depigmented and lighter in color than the surrounding retina
◆ Geographic atrophy (**Fig. 40.3**)—confluent area of RPE and choriocapillary atrophy, typically occurring at macula. Geographic atrophy appears as a depigmented area overlying visible large choroidal vessels.
◆ Peripheral reticular pigmentary changes

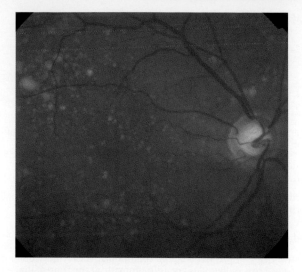

Fig. 40.1 Drusen—multiple, nonrefractile, yellow subretinal deposits with indistinct margins in nonexudative "dry" age-related macular degeneration.

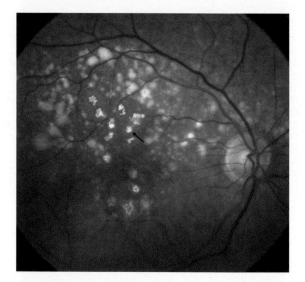

Fig. 40.2 Multiple, nonrefractile, yellow subretinal deposits with indistinct margins representing drusen. Calcified drusen (*arrow*) are refractile, white-yellow deposits and may be mistaken for hard exudates.

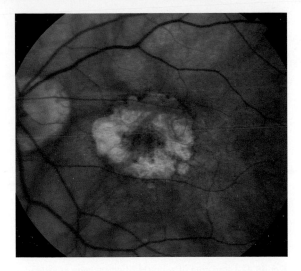

Fig. 40.3 Geographic atrophy—patchy area of hypopigmentation with visible large choroidal vessels indicates loss of retinal pigment epithelium and choriocapillaries in this patient with nonexudative "dry" age-related macular degeneration. Pigment clumping is also present.

Exudative ("Wet")

Exudative AMD is characterized by development of choroidal neovascularization (CNV) extending into the sub-RPE and subretinal spaces. Leakage of plasma or blood from CNV results in serous or hemorrhagic macular elevation. Symptoms include acute or subacute loss or distortion of central vision, central scotoma, and photopsia. Changes of exudative AMD are primarily located within the macular region.

Fundus Features

◆ Subretinal/choroidal neovascular complex—a gray-brown lesion located deep to the retina. It may be associated with surrounding brown pigmentation (sign of chronicity) or hemorrhage (sign of activity).
◆ Subretinal or intraretinal hemorrhage (**Fig. 40.4**)
◆ Subretinal fluid—neurosensory retinal elevation
◆ Subretinal hard exudates—late feature
◆ Retinal pigment epithelial detachment (PED)—a blister-like elevation of RPE
◆ Accompanying changes of "dry" AMD (e.g., drusen, pigment clumping, geographic atrophy)
◆ Subretinal fibrosis (**Fig. 40.5**)—irregular gray-white lesion in the subretinal space. It represents later stages of "wet" AMD. When the subretinal fibrosis is extensive, with significant loss of vision, it is termed disciform scar (end-stage AMD).

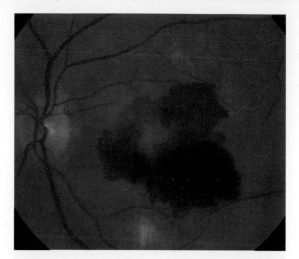

Fig. 40.4 Large area of subretinal hemorrhage in exudative "wet" age-related macular degeneration. The retinal vessels can be seen passing over (internal to) the hemorrhage.

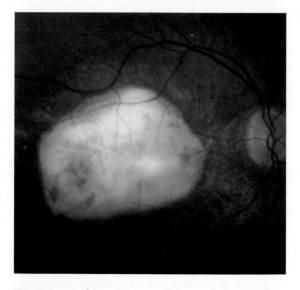

Fig. 40.5 Disciform scar—gray-white area of subretinal fibrosis affecting the central macular region in advanced exudative "wet" age-related macular degeneration.

◆ Choroidal (Subretinal) Neovascularization

Choroidal neovascularization is the development of abnormal neovascular complexes originating from choriocapillaries (**Fig. 40.6**). The vascular complexes grow into the sub-RPE and subretinal spaces. Abnormal vascular permeability results in leakage of serum into these spaces. The subsequent accumulation of subretinal or sub-RPE fluid causes distortion and loss of vision. Abnormally fragile CNV complexes may bleed, causing submacular hemorrhage and severe loss of vision.

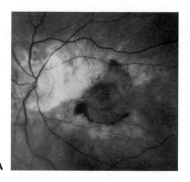 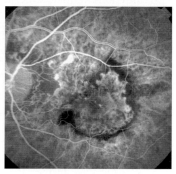

A   B

Fig. 40.6 Choroidal neovascularization (CNV). (**A**) Area of choroidal neovascular membrane with overlying hyperpigmentation and surrounding thin rim of subretinal hemorrhage. (**B**) Fundus fluorescein angiogram showing the choroidal neovascular complex. The surrounding hypofluorescent (dark) area corresponds to subretinal hemorrhage.

Conditions Associated with Choroidal Neovascularization

- ◆ Age-related macular degeneration
- ◆ Myopic degeneration
- ◆ Angioid streaks
- ◆ Best disease
- ◆ Fundus flavimaculatus
- ◆ Optic nerve drusen
- ◆ Ocular histoplasmosis syndrome
- ◆ Multifocal choroiditis
- ◆ Serpiginous choroidopathy
- ◆ Toxoplasmosis
- ◆ Toxocariasis
- ◆ Rubella
- ◆ Vogt-Koyanagi-Harada syndrome
- ◆ Behçet syndrome
- ◆ Sympathetic ophthalmia
- ◆ Choroidal nevus
- ◆ Choroidal tumors
- ◆ Traumatic choroidal rupture
- ◆ Laser photocoagulation of retina
- ◆ Idiopathic

◆ Retinal Detachment

Retinal detachment is caused by the accumulation of fluid within the subretinal space, causing separation and elevation of the neurosensory retina from the underlying retinal pigment epithelium, which remains attached to the wall of the eye. Retinal detachment is categorized into rhegmatogenous, tractional, exudative, and combined tractional/rhegmatogenous types, based on underlying pathogenic mechanisms. All forms of retinal detachment can cause progressive painless loss of vision.

Rhegmatogenous Retinal Detachment

Rhegmatogenous retinal detachment (RRD) is characterized by the presence of a retinal break, which allows entry of fluid from the vitreous cavity into the subretinal space. Symptoms include painless loss of vision, flashes, floaters, and visual field defect.

Fundus Features

◆ Retinal break (**Figs. 40.7 and 40.8**)—usually in the peripheral retina; may be solitary or multiple
◆ Convex elevation of the retina
◆ Mobile retina
◆ Irregular surface
◆ Corrugation lines (**Fig. 40.9**)
◆ Typically starts in the periphery around a retinal break and extends both anteriorly to the ora serrata and posteriorly toward the macula

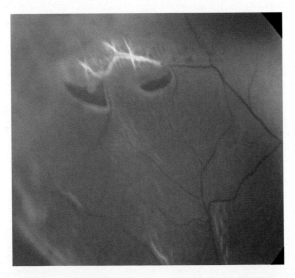

Fig. 40.7 Rhegmatogenous retinal detachment with "horseshoe" tears adjacent to an area of lattice degeneration.

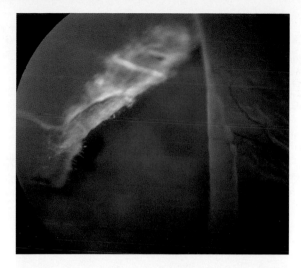

Fig. 40.8 Rhegmatogenous retinal detachment with a giant retinal tear adjacent to an area of lattice degeneration.

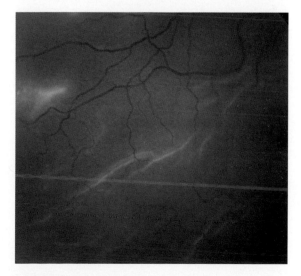

Fig. 40.9 Rhegmatogenous retinal detachment. The retina is slightly opaque, the vessels are seen curving forward, and corrugation lines are present. The choroidal color and vessels are not visible.

Causes

Causes of RRD include conditions that are associated with retinal breaks:

◆ Posterior vitreous detachment
◆ Trauma
◆ Peripheral retinal degenerations and atrophic retinal holes
◆ Retinal necrosis
◆ Severe vitreoretinal traction

Tractional Retinal Detachment

Tractional retinal detachment (TRD) is caused by contraction of membranes and bands that form on the surface of the retina, across the vitreous cavity (**Fig. 40.10**), or in the subretinal space. Contraction of these membranes and bands pulls the neurosensory retina away from the RPE, resulting in a localized retinal detachment.

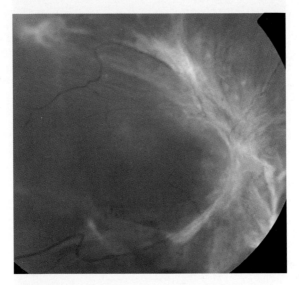

Fig. 40.10 Tractional retinal detachment with extensive fibrovascular proliferation in a patient with advanced diabetic eye disease.

Fundus Features

◆ Smooth concave surface
◆ Presence of vitreoretinal traction bands and membranes
◆ Absence of retinal break
◆ No retinal mobility
◆ Usually located posterior to the equator
◆ Rarely extends to the ora serrata

Conditions Associated with Tractional Retinal Detachment

See Chapter 17, Retinal Detachment

Serous/Exudative Retinal Detachment

Exudative retinal detachment occurs as a result of impairment of inner or outer blood–retinal barriers, which are at the level of the retinal capillary endothelium and the RPE, respectively. When the blood–retinal barrier is damaged, fluid can leak into the subretinal space. Some of the fluid is actively transported across the RPE into the choriocapillary system. As this mechanism becomes saturated, there is accumulation of fluid between the neurosensory retina and the RPE, resulting in an exudative/serous retinal detachment. Impairment of blood–retinal barriers may arise from inflammatory processes, abnormal intra- and extravascular osmotic pressures, structural and functional anomalies of the retinal and choroidal vasculatures, and trauma.

Symptoms include blurred vision, metamorphopsia, micropsia, and relative scotoma.

Fundus Features

◆ Retinal elevation
◆ Smooth surface
◆ Absence of a retinal break
◆ Shifting subretinal fluid—changes in the location and the shape of the retinal detachment in accordance with the patient's position

Conditions Associated with Exudative/Serous Retinal Detachment

See Chapter 17, Retinal Detachment

◆ Retinitis Pigmentosa

Retinitis pigmentosa (RP) is a group of inherited retinal dystrophies with diffuse impairment of photoreceptor and pigment epithelium function. RP is characterized by night blindness, progressive loss of peripheral vision, pigmentary retinopathy, and abnormal electroretinography (ERG). Central vision may become affected in later stages of the disease. Inheritance may be X-linked, autosomal recessive, or autosomal dominant.

Fundus Features (Figs. 40.11 and 40.12)

◆ Diffuse bone-spicule pigment clumping—Pigmentary changes may be minimal in some cases.
◆ Retinal arteriolar attenuation
◆ Waxy pallor of the optic disc
◆ Macular pigmentary change
◆ Cystoid macular edema (in up to 20–30% of cases)
◆ Vitreous cells and debris

Other Ocular Features

◆ Posterior subcapsular cataract
◆ Abnormal ERG, electro-oculography (EOG)

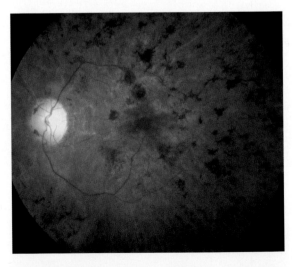

Fig. 40.11   Retinitis pigmentosa. Extensive bone-spicule pigmentation, diffuse retinal pigment epithelial atrophy, waxy pallor of the optic disc, and attenuated blood vessels are characteristic findings.

Fig. 40.12   Typical bone-spicule pigment clumping in retinitis pigmentosa.

Systemic Disorders Associated with Retinitis Pigmentosa

◆ Refsum disease—RP, optic atrophy, neurosensory hearing loss, cerebellar ataxia, ichthyosis, elevated serum phytanic acid
◆ Abetalipoproteinemia—RP, malabsorption, hypovitaminosis A and E, neuropathy, cerebellar dysfunction
◆ Kearns-Sayre syndrome—atypical RP, external ophthalmoplegia, ptosis, heart block
◆ Alström syndrome—RP, deafness, obesity, baldness, diabetes mellitus, cardiomyopathy, acanthosis nigricans, hypogonadism
◆ Bardet-Biedl syndrome—RP, obesity, hypogonadism, mental retardation, polydactyly
◆ Alagille syndrome—RP, posterior embryotoxon, neonatal jaundice, pulmonary valve stenosis, arterial stenosis, abnormal vertebrae and facies
◆ Cockayne syndrome—RP, dwarfism, deafness, premature senility, mental retardation, intracranial calcification
◆ Friedreich ataxia—RP, optic atrophy, spinocerebellar degeneration, incoordination, neurosensory hearing loss
◆ Olivopontocerebellar atrophy—RP, macular atrophy, external ophthalmoplegia, cerebellar ataxia
◆ Usher syndrome—RP, neurosensory hearing loss, problems with balance (ataxia)
◆ Mevalonic aciduria—RP, psychomotor retardation

Differential Diagnosis of Pigmentary Retinopathy

◆ RP—isolated or in association with systemic syndromes
◆ Congenital rubella
◆ Syphilis—congenital, acquired
◆ Resolved retinal detachment
◆ Resolved choroidal hemorrhage
◆ Severe blunt trauma
◆ Ophthalmic artery occlusion—late stages
◆ Vogt-Koyanagi-Harada disease (**Fig. 40.13**)
◆ Panretinal laser photocoagulation scars
◆ Drug-related retinopathy

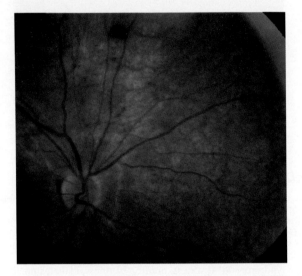

Fig. 40.13 Differential diagnosis of pigmentary retinopathy includes prior serous retinal detachment or choroidal detachment. Extensive pigmentary retinopathy is present in this patient with resolved serous retinal detachment from Vogt-Koyanagi-Harada disease.

◆ Macular Hole

Macular hole is a round, full-thickness defect in the central macula. Idiopathic macular hole occurs primarily in the sixth and seventh decades of life and affects women more frequently than men (3:1). Symptoms include painless loss of central vision (20/40–20/400), and central distortion.

Fundus Features (Fig. 40.14)

◆ Round defect (⅛ to ⅓ disc diameter [DD]) in center of macula
◆ Surrounding cuff of shallow subretinal fluid
◆ Small yellow deposits within the hole
◆ Operculum within the vitreous cavity overlying the hole
◆ Epiretinal membrane

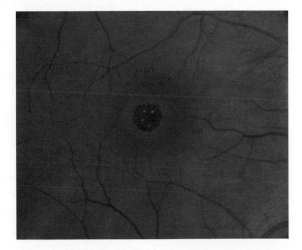

Fig. 40.14 Idiopathic macular hole with thin cuff of subretinal fluid and small yellow deposits in the bed of the hole.

Stages of Macular Hole

- Stage 1—foveal cyst
- Stage 2—full-thickness hole <400 μm
- Stage 3—full-thickness hole ≥400 μm, no posterior vitreous detachment
- Stage 4—full-thickness hole, posterior vitreous detachment

Conditions Associated with Macular Hole

- Idiopathic macular hole
- Blunt ocular trauma
- Pathologic myopia
- Epiretinal membrane
- Retinal detachment surgery
- Other intraocular surgeries
- Inadvertent YAG laser injury

Pseudomacular hole has the ophthalmoscopic appearance of an apparent macular hole, but it results from the distortion of the surrounding macular area by a translucent or opaque epiretinal membrane. Pseudomacular hole does not represent a full-thickness defect in the retina.

Lamellar hole represents a partial-thickness retinal defect in the central macular region. Pseudomacular hole and lamellar hole may be difficult to differentiate from full-thickness macular hole by ophthalmoscopy alone. Optical coherence tomography (OCT) is useful for accurate diagnosis.

◆ Pathologic Myopia

Pathologic or high myopia is arbitrarily defined as myopic refractive error greater than 6.5 diopters or an axial length greater than 26 mm.

Symptoms

- Severe nearsightedness
- Painless loss of vision
  - Choroidal neovascularization in macular region
  - Geographic myopic degeneration, lacquer cracks
  - Retinal detachment
  - Cataract
- Image minification
- Impaired stereopsis
- Impaired color vision
- Impaired dark adaptation
- Visual field abnormalities—scotoma, enlarged blind spot
- Amblyopia

Fundus Features (Figs. 40.15 and 40.16)

- ◆ Temporal peripapillary crescent
- ◆ Tilting of optic disc
- ◆ Peripapillary chorioretinal atrophy
- ◆ Straightening of retinal vessels
- ◆ Posterior staphyloma
- ◆ Pigment epithelial mottling
- ◆ Geographic and gyrate areas of RPE and choriocapillary atrophy
- ◆ Prominent, visible choroidal vessels
- ◆ Lacquer cracks
- ◆ Isolated, focal subretinal hemorrhages
- ◆ Fuchs spots—focal RPE hyperplasia in macular region
- ◆ Choroidal neovascularization
- ◆ Foveal schisis, foveal cyst
- ◆ Lamellar macular hole
- ◆ Full-thickness macular hole
- ◆ Localized posterior pole retinal detachment
- ◆ Peripheral focal or diffuse chorioretinal atrophy
- ◆ Peripheral retinal degeneration—lattice, "cobblestone," microcystic degenerations. Peripheral retinoschisis is not a feature of myopic degeneration.
- ◆ Peripheral retinal breaks—hole, "horseshoe" tear, giant retinal tear
- ◆ Rhegmatogenous retinal detachment
- ◆ Spontaneous, traumatic, or surgically induced choroidal hemorrhage
- ◆ Vitreous syneresis
- ◆ Posterior vitreous detachment (PVD)

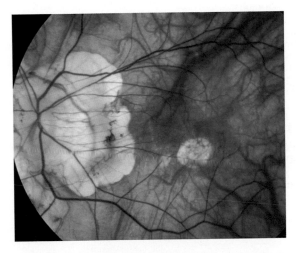

Fig. 40.15 Myopic degeneration. Characteristic peripapillary atrophy, straightening of the temporal disc vessels, visible choroidal vessels, lacquer cracks, and geographic atrophy are present.

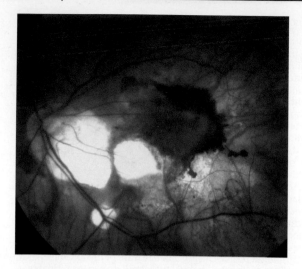

Fig. 40.16 Subretinal hemorrhage due to choroidal neovascularization (CNV) in a patient with myopic degeneration.

Other Ophthalmic Features

◆ Large thin cornea
◆ Deep anterior chamber
◆ Posterior subcapsular lens opacity
◆ Glaucoma—primary open angle, pigment dispersion glaucoma, normal tension glaucoma
◆ Scleral thinning
◆ Pseudoproptosis

Systemic Associations of Pathologic Myopia

◆ Marfan syndrome
◆ Ehlers-Danlos syndrome
◆ Stickler syndrome
◆ Prematurity

Pearls

- Macular drusen may superficially resemble hard exudates. In the setting of diabetic retinopathy, this resemblance may cause diagnostic confusion. It is important to distinguish these entities, because drusen are typically not visually significant, whereas the presence of hard exudates in the macular region indicates significant vascular retinopathy, such as diabetic or hypertensive retinopathy. The following characteristics help distinguish between the two entities.

Hard Exudates	Drusen
Bright yellow	Dull yellow or cream colored
Intraretinal	Subretinal
Refractile	Nonrefractile,* dull
Sharp borders	Poorly defined borders
Associated features of vascular retinopathy	Associated features of AMD

* Regressing, calcified drusen may appear refractile.

- The most common cause of subretinal hemorrhage in the macular region is exudative AMD. It is important to distinguish subretinal hemorrhage from other forms of fundus hemorrhage, because subretinal hemorrhage in the macula typically signifies exudative AMD with its risk of severe visual loss. Diagnosis of subretinal hemorrhage can be aided by the following:
  - Patchy configuration of the hemorrhage, often with irregular borders
  - Variable size
  - Visibility of retinal blood vessels overlying (internal to) the area of hemorrhage

Appendix A: Abbreviations of Retinal Terminology

AIDS:	acquired immunodeficiency syndrome
AION:	anterior ischemic optic neuropathy
AMD:	age-related macular degeneration
BCVA:	best-corrected visual acuity
BGDR (BDR):	background diabetic retinopathy
BRAO:	branch retinal artery occlusion
BRVO:	branch retinal vein occlusion
CF:	count fingers; a crude measure of vision in severe visual loss
CME:	cystoid macular edema
CNV:	choroidal neovascularization (also see SRNVM)
CRAO:	central retinal artery occlusion
CRVO:	central retinal vein occlusion
CSME:	clinically significant macular edema
CSR:	central serous chorioretinopathy
CWS:	cotton-wool spot
DA:	disc area; unit of area corresponding to the size of the optic disc
DD:	disc diameter; diameter of the optic disc, ~1700 μm
DME:	diabetic macular edema
DR:	diabetic retinopathy
EOG:	electro-oculogram
ERG:	electro-retinogram
FFA:	fundus fluorescein angiogram
GRT:	giant retinal tear
HIV:	human immunodeficiency virus
HM:	hand motion, hand movement; a measure of vision in severe visual loss
HST:	horseshoe tear
ICP:	intracranial pressure
IOP:	intraocular pressure
IRH:	intraretinal hemorrhage
KP:	keratic precipitate
LP:	light perception
LVA:	low-vision aid
ME:	macular edema
MH:	macular hole
NLP:	no light perception
NPDR:	nonproliferative diabetic retinopathy
NVD:	neovascularization at the optic disc
NVE:	neovascularization elsewhere in the retina
NVG:	neovascular glaucoma

NVI:	neovascularization of iris (rubeosis iris)
OCT:	optical coherence tomography
OD:	right eye, *oculus dexter*
OS:	left eye, *oculus sinister*
OU:	both eyes, *oculus uterque*
PDR:	proliferative diabetic retinopathy
PED:	pigment epithelial detachment
PPL:	pars plana lensectomy
PPV:	pars plana vitrectomy
PRP:	panretinal laser photocoagulation
PVD:	posterior vitreous detachment
PVR:	proliferative vitreoretinopathy
RAPD:	relative afferent pupillary defect
RD:	retinal detachment
ROP:	retinopathy of prematurity
RP:	retinitis pigmentosa
RPE:	retinal pigment epithelium
RRD:	rhegmatogenous retinal detachment
SRF:	subretinal fluid
SRH:	subretinal hemorrhage
SRNVM:	subretinal neovascular membrane (also see CNV)
TRD:	tractional retinal detachment
VA:	visual acuity
VEGF:	vascular endothelial growth factor
VEP:	visual evoked potential
VER:	visual evoked response
VF:	visual field
VH:	vitreous hemorrhage

Appendix B: Glossary of Retinal Terminology

Amaurosis fugax: transient loss of vision lasting a few minutes, due to transient retinal arteriolar occlusion by emboli

Amblyopia: reduction of best-corrected visual acuity in the absence of organic lesions. Amblyopia most frequently results from childhood strabismus or asymmetric refractive errors.

Chemosis: edema of conjunctiva

Coloboma: congenital absence of any eye or eyelid structure

Diopter (D): unit of refractive power

Diplopia: double vision

Disc diameter (DD): diameter of the optic disc, ~1700 μm. DD is a useful unit of measuring retinal lesion size by comparing the lesion to the size of the optic disc.

Episcleritis: inflammation of the episclera, the tissue between the conjunctiva and the sclera

Exophthalmos: protrusion of the eye relative to the orbital rim, often due to thyroid eye disease

Fluorescein angiography: a diagnostic test utilizing intravenous injection of fluorescein dye. Photographs of the retina and choroid are taken with special filters, evaluating the integrity of the retinal and choroidal blood vessels and adjacent tissues.

Fovea: the central part of the macula, corresponding to the central vision. Fovea measures ~1.5 mm in diameter.

Foveola the central 0.35 mm of the fovea

Hyperopia: farsightedness

Hyphema: presence of blood in the anterior chamber

Hypopyon: layering of white blood cells in the anterior chamber

Hypotony: abnormally low intraocular pressure (<6 mm Hg)

Iritis: anterior uveitis; inflammation of the iris and anterior chamber

Juxtafoveal: adjacent to the fovea

Juxtapapillary: adjacent to the optic disc

Keratic precipitates (KP): focal inflammatory deposits on the endothelial surface of the cornea seen in anterior uveitis

Macula: area of the retina centered over the posterior pole of the fundus, measuring ~5 disc diameters, bordered by the optic disc nasally and the temporal vascular arcades superiorly and inferiorly

Metamorphopsia: abnormal visual perception causing objects to appear distorted

Microphthalmia: congenitally small eye, often with disorganized internal structures

Micropsia: abnormal visual perception causing objects to appear smaller than normal

Miosis: constriction of pupil

Mydriasis: dilation of pupil

Myopia: nearsightedness

Nanophthalmos: a congenitally small eye with formed internal structures

Nerve fiber layer: the innermost (most superficial layer) of retina, containing the nerve fibers originating in the ganglion cell layer. These fibers form the optic nerve, partly decussate in the optic chiasm, and terminate at the lateral geniculate ganglion.

Nyctalopia: difficulty seeing at night; night blindness

Ora serrata: junction of the peripheral retina and the pars plana

Papillary: related to the optic disc

Parafoveal: a 0.5-mm-wide ring surrounding the fovea

Pars plana: flattened posterior portion of the ciliary body. Posteriorly, it ends at ora serrata (the junction of pars plana and the retina).

Perifoveal: a 1.5-mm-wide ring surrounding the parafoveal zone

Peripapillary: surrounding the optic disc

Photophobia: sensitivity to light; ocular pain on exposure to light

Photopsia: visual sensation of flashes of light

Poliosis: whitening of the eyelashes

Posterior vitreous detachment (PVD): separation of the posterior cortical vitreous from the retina. PVD is usually a physiologic, age-related phenomenon associated with liquefaction (syneresis) of the vitreous. PVD can cause symptoms of floaters and flashes of light, and occasionally leads to vitreous hemorrhage, retinal tear, and retinal detachment.

Prepapillary: overlying the optic disc, internal to the optic disc

Presbyopia: age-related decrease in the ability to accommodate and see clearly at near distances.

Proptosis: protrusion of the eye relative to the orbital rim due to orbital disease

Relative afferent pupillary defect (RAPD): a relative decrease in pupillary constriction in one eye when compared with the other eye, using the swinging-flashlight test. RAPD usually indicates asymmetric optic nerve disease.

Retinoschisis: splitting of the retinal neurosensory layers

Scotoma area of relative or absolute visual loss in the visual field

Staphyloma: bulging of the eye wall and its layers. Posterior staphyloma is usually associated with severe myopia and is associated with thinning of the sclera, choroid, and retina in the affected area

Stereopsis: binocular depth perception

Strabismus: misalignment of the two eyes

Subfoveal: deep to (under) the fovea

Syneresis: liquefaction of the vitreous gel; usually a physiologic age-related phenomenon

Uveitis: inflammation of the uveal tissue. Anterior uveitis (iritis) is inflammation manifesting primarily in the iris and anterior chamber. In intermediate uveitis, the inflammation is predominantly in the anterior vitreous and the pars plana. In posterior uveitis, the inflammation mainly affects the choroid and posterior vitreous. The term *panuveitis* is used to describe intraocular inflammation affecting all segments of the eye

Vitritis: inflammation of the vitreous, characterized by the presence of inflammatory cells within the vitreous, visible on biomicroscopic examination

Index

Note: Page numbers followed by *f* and *t* indicate figures and tables, respectively.

Conditions Associated with a Hypercoagulable State

◆ Inherited
  ◦ Factor V Leiden
  ◦ Prothrombin 20210A mutation
  ◦ Antithrombin III deficiency
  ◦ Protein C deficiency
  ◦ Protein S deficiency
  ◦ Heparin cofactor II deficiency
  ◦ Primary hyperhomocystinemia*
  ◦ Dysfibrinogenemia
  ◦ Defects in fibrinolysis
◆ Acquired
  ◦ Anticardiolipin antibody syndrome
  ◦ Dysfibrinogenemia (liver disease)
  ◦ Acquired hyperhomocystinemia*
  ◦ Medications (chemotherapeutic medications)
  ◦ Heparin-induced thrombopathy
  ◦ Pregnancy/postpartum
  ◦ Estrogen administration (oral contraceptives)
  ◦ Malignant disease
  ◦ Myeloproliferative disorders
  ◦ Paroxysmal nocturnal hemoglobinuria
  ◦ Hyperviscosity
  ◦ Chronic inflammatory disease
  ◦ Disseminated intravascular coagulation (DIC)
  ◦ Chronic congestive heart disease
  ◦ Nephrotic syndrome
  ◦ Severe dehydration

*Some medical authorities do not believe that hyperhomocystinemia causes a hypercoaguable state.

◆ Bleeding Disorders

Hypocoagulable states predispose to bleeding.

Fundus Features

◆ Retinal hemorrhages
  ◦ Flame-shaped—most common type of hemorrhage
  ◦ Dot and blot
  ◦ Preretinal
◆ Retrohyaloid/subhyaloid hemorrhage
◆ Vitreous hemorrhage
◆ Subretinal hemorrhage
◆ Choroidal hemorrhage
◆ Optic disc hemorrhage

Other Ophthalmic Features

- ◆ Orbital hemorrhage
- ◆ Eyelid ecchymosis
- ◆ Subconjunctival hemorrhage
- ◆ Neuro-ophthalmic
  - ○ Visual field defects
  - ○ Internuclear ophthalmoplegia
  - ○ Cranial nerve palsies

Conditions Associated with Bleeding Disorders

- ◆ Clotting factor abnormalities
  - ○ Inherited
    - ◆ Hemophilia (factor VIII deficiency)
    - ◆ Christmas disease
    - ◆ Von Willebrand's disease
  - ○ Acquired
    - ◆ Liver disease
    - ◆ Vitamin K deficiency
    - ◆ Heparin/Warfarin administration
- ◆ Platelet count or function abnormalities
  - ○ Thrombocytopenia
  - ○ Hermansky-Pudlak syndrome—thrombocytopenia associated with oculocutaneous albinism
  - ○ Aspirin/dipyridamole/clopidogrel administration
- ◆ Mixed clotting factors and platelet abnormality
- ◆ Disseminated Intravascular Coagulation
- ◆ Blood transfusion

◆ Disseminated Intravascular Coagulation (DIC)

In DIC both thrombotic and hemorrhagic phenomena occur simultaneously. Retina and choroid can be affected by embolic, thrombotic, and hemorrhagic processes.

Fundus Features

- ◆ Retinal hemorrhages
  - ○ Superficial flame-shaped
  - ○ Dot and blot
  - ○ White-centered (pseudo-Roth spots)
- ◆ Subretinal hemorrhage
- ◆ Choroidal hemorrhage
- ◆ Cotton-wool spots
- ◆ Retinal vascular occlusion
- ◆ Serous retinal detachment
- ◆ Choroidal ischemia and infarcts—During the acute phase, this manifests as creamy-yellow, placoid subretinal/choroidal lesions. Overlying serous retinal detachment may be present. Later, these lesions become pigmented atrophic scars.
- ◆ Vitreous hemorrhage
- ◆ Optic disc swelling

◆ Anemia

Retinal hemorrhages occur in severe anemia (Hb <8 g/100 mL). Anemic patients who also have thrombocytopenia are more likely to have retinal hemorrhages. Retinal neovascularization may occur in severe chronic anemia.

Fundus Features

◆ Retinal hemorrhages
  ○ Flame-shaped
  ○ Dot and blot
  ○ White-centered (pseudo-Roth spots)
◆ Microaneurysms
◆ Cotton-wool spots (**Fig. 30.12**)
◆ Retinal edema
◆ Hard exudates
◆ Neovascularization
◆ Optic nerve
  ○ Papilledema
  ○ Ischemic optic neuropathy
  ○ Optic atrophy

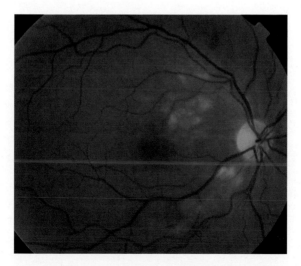

Fig. 30.12 Cotton-wool spots and faint retinal hemorrhages in a patient with severe anemia.

Pearls

- Severe cases of hyperviscosity retinopathy may resemble central retinal vein occlusion (i.e., "blood and thunder" appearance). However, hyperviscosity retinopathy is usually bilateral, and changes resolve once blood viscosity is normalized.

31 Gastrointestinal Disorders

◆ Inflammatory Bowel Disease

Inflammatory bowel disease may be associated with ocular inflammation, infiltration, and secondary infections.

Fundus Features

- ◆ Retinal hemorrhages
- ◆ Retinal edema
- ◆ Hard exudates
- ◆ Vascular sheathing (**Fig. 31.1**)
- ◆ Vascular occlusion
- ◆ Serous retinal detachment
- ◆ Retinal infiltrates
- ◆ Chorioretinal infiltrates
- ◆ Endogenous endophthalmitis—bacteremia/fungemia
- ◆ Optic disc edema—optic neuritis
- ◆ Vitritis

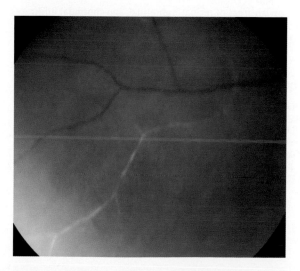

Fig. 31.1 Vascular sheathing in a patient with Crohn disease. The fundus view is hazy due to the presence of vitritis.

Other Ophthalmic Features

◆ Decreased vision
◆ Night blindness—vitamin A deficiency
◆ Episcleritis
◆ Scleritis
◆ Scleromalacia
◆ Corneal infiltrates/keratitis
◆ Uveitis—anterior and posterior
◆ Orbital myositis
◆ Dacryoadenitis

◆ Whipple Disease

Whipple disease is a multisystem condition caused by *Tropheryma whippleii*. It is characterized by fever, abdominal pain, steatorrhea, arthritis, polyserositis, and various central nervous system manifestations.

Fundus Features

◆ Retinal hemorrhages
◆ Cotton-wool spots
◆ Retinal vascular sheathing—represents vasculitis
◆ Retinal vascular occlusion
◆ Small yellowish areas of retinal, subretinal, and choroidal infiltrates
◆ Optic disc edema
◆ Vitreous opacities

Other Ophthalmic Features

◆ Conjunctival edema (chemosis)
◆ Scleritis/episcleritis
◆ Corneal infiltrates/keratitis
◆ Uveitis—anterior and posterior
◆ Neuro-ophthalmic
  ◦ Gaze palsy
  ◦ Nystagmus
  ◦ Ptosis

◆ Familial Adenomatous Polyposis (Gardner Syndrome)

Familial adenomatous polyposis is an autosomal dominant condition, characterized by intestinal polyposis with high prevalence of adenocarcinoma by age 50.

Fundus Features

◆ Multiple (>4), bilateral, cigar-shaped, or ovoid foci of flattened retinal pigment epithelial hypertrophy similar to lesions seen in congenital hypertrophy of retinal pigment epithelium (CHRPE) (**Fig. 31.2**). These are flat darkly pigmented lesions, often with areas of hypopigmentation, ranging from 0.1 to 10 mm in size. Multifocal CHRPEs are an important congenital phenotypic marker for patients with familial adenomatous polyposis.

Systemic Features

◆ Intestinal polyposis
◆ Adenocarcinoma of colon
◆ Thyroid carcinoma
◆ Osteomas of skull, facial, and orbital bones
◆ Epidermoid cysts
◆ Teeth abnormalities

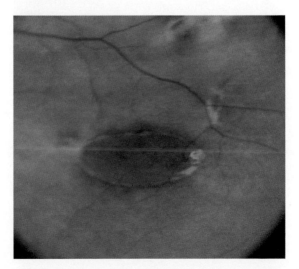

Fig. 31.2 Familial adenomatous polyposis—ovoid, cigar-shaped flat pigmented area of retinal pigment epithelial hypertrophy in a patient with familial adenomatous polyposis.

◆ Pancreatitis

Pancreatitis may result in a microvascular retinopathy through several mechanisms, including microembolization of adipose tissue, complement-induced leukocyte aggregates, platelet aggregates, and fibrin.

Fundus Features

◆ Purtscher-like retinopathy (**Fig. 31.3**)
  ◆ Purtscher-like retinopathy is usually a self-limiting condition with little serious visual consequence. It is characterized by:
    ◦ Multiple cotton-wool spots
    ◦ Superficial flame-shaped hemorrhages
    ◦ Retinal edema
◆ Serous retinal detachment
◆ Retinal vascular occlusion (**Fig. 31.4**)
◆ Choroidal ischemia/infarct
◆ Optic disc edema

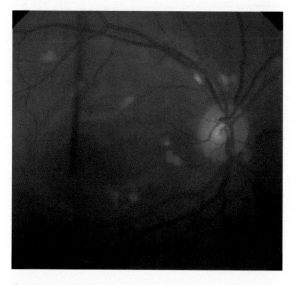

Fig. 31.3 Mild Purtscher-like retinopathy with multiple cotton-wool spots in a patient with acute pancreatitis.

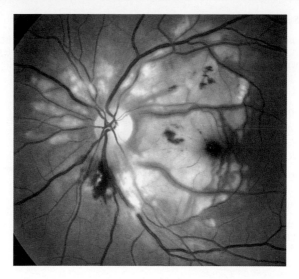

Fig. 31.4 Severe Purtscher-like retinopathy in a patient with acute necrotizing pancreatitis. Multiple cotton-wool spots, retinal hemorrhages, and large areas of cloudy swelling of the retina (due to vascular occlusions) are present.

◆ Liver Disease

Chronic Liver Failure

Chronic liver failure may be associated with increased bleeding tendencies, anemia, and various nutritional deficiencies, such as vitamin A deficiency. Treatment with interferon α may cause retinopathy.

Fundus Features

- ◆ Retinal hemorrhages
- ◆ Cotton-wool spots
- ◆ Diffuse peripheral pigmentary changes/mottling
- ◆ Interferon-associated retinopathy

Other Ophthalmic Features

- ◆ Nyctalopia
- ◆ Dry eye sensation
- ◆ White, keratinized conjunctival plaques—Bitot's spots
- ◆ Corneal ulceration

Alagille Syndrome

Alagille syndrome is a rare familial condition characterized by chronic intrahepatic cholestasis with paucity of intrahepatic bile ducts, pulmonary artery stenosis, triangular facies, and renal and neurologic abnormalities.

Fundus Features

◆ Pigmentary retinopathy
◆ Choroidal folds
◆ Anomalous optic disc

Other Ophthalmic Features

◆ Posterior embryotoxon
◆ Axenfeld's anomaly
◆ Band keratopathy
◆ Ectopic pupil
◆ Strabismus
◆ Myopia

Pearls

- Presence of multiple cigar-shaped or ovoid flat pigmented fundus lesions (similar to CHRPE lesions) is a useful congenital phenotypic marker for patients with familial adenomatous polyposis.

- Interferon α, when used for the treatment of chronic hepatitis, may cause retinopathy. Interferon-associated retinopathy is usually an asymptomatic, self-limiting, and transient condition, not requiring discontinuation of interferon therapy.

◆ Sarcoidosis

Sarcoidosis is a chronic granulomatous systemic disease of unknown etiology. Histopathologically, it is characterized by noncaseating granulomatous infiltrations. In young adults, sarcoidosis tends to present with acute symptoms (e.g., erythema nodosum, arthritis, and acute uveitis). In older patients it has a more chronic presentation (e.g., interstitial lung disease, chronic arthritis, and chronic uveitis). Sarcoidosis occurs most commonly in the African-American population.

Twenty-five percent of patients with sarcoidosis have ocular involvement. Eighty-five percent of patients with ocular sarcoidosis have abnormal computed tomography (CT) of the chest.

Fundus Features

◆ Periphlebitis/vascular sheathing (**Figs. 32.1 and 32.2**)
◆ "Candle-wax" exudates—focal yellow-white perivascular exudates
◆ Retinal infiltrates—multiple, focal yellow-white lesions of varying size. More commonly seen in the inferior retina (**Fig. 32.3**)
◆ Choroidal infiltrates—solitary or multiple yellowish subretinal lesions that may be slightly elevated (**Fig. 32.4**)
◆ Venous occlusion
◆ Retinal neovascularization—peripheral fan-shaped neovascular complexes
◆ Macular edema
◆ Epiretinal membrane
◆ Vitreous infiltrates—white, fluffy opacities in inferior vitreous that may appear as "snowballs" or "strings of pearls"
◆ Vitritis—inflammatory cells in the vitreous
◆ Vitreous hemorrhage
◆ Atrophic chorioretinal scars—variable size, pigmented or depigmented, more frequently involve the inferior fundus. Chorioretinal scars are rarely associated with choroidal neovascularization.
◆ Optic nerve granuloma (**Fig. 32.5**)
◆ Optic disc neovascularization
◆ Optic disc swelling
  ◦ Papilledema—secondary to neurosarcoidosis
  ◦ Optic neuritis
  ◦ Chronic uveitis

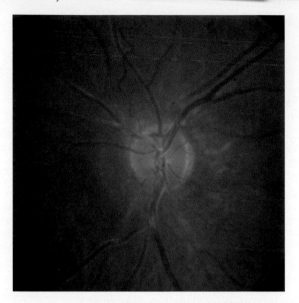

Fig. 32.1 Vascular sheathing of the retinal veins and arteries in a patient with sarcoidosis.

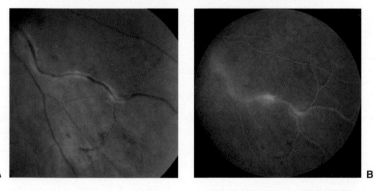

A   B

Fig. 32.2 Retinal periphlebitis. **(A)** Segmental perivenous cuffing and infiltration, as well as retinal hemorrhages in a patient with sarcoidosis. **(B)** Fundus fluorescein angiogram showing segmental staining of the venous wall characteristic of periphlebitis.

Fig. 32.3 Sarcoidosis—vitreous and retinal infiltrates in a patient with panuveitis and sarcoidosis. The view of the retina is hazy due to the presence of vitritis.

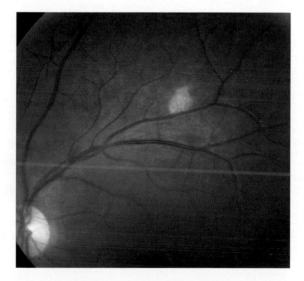

Fig. 32.4 Old chorioretinal infiltrate and vitritis in a patient with panuveitis and sarcoidosis.

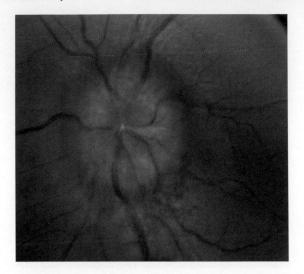

Fig. 32.5   Sarcoid infiltration of the optic nerve. The optic disc is elevated and hyperemic and has blurred margins.

Other Ophthalmic Features

- ◆ Symptoms
  - ◦ Blurred vision
  - ◦ Floaters
  - ◦ Redness
  - ◦ Photophobia
  - ◦ Ocular pain
  - ◦ Dry-eye symptoms
  - ◦ Asymptomatic
- ◆ Eyelid—lupus pernio, millet seed lesions
- ◆ Lacrimal gland infiltration
- ◆ Keratoconjunctivitis sicca
- ◆ Conjunctival infiltration/granulomas
- ◆ Episcleritis/scleritis
- ◆ Anterior uveitis—"mutton-fat" keratic precipitates
- ◆ Iris nodules—Busacca (iris stroma) and Koeppe (pupil margin) nodules
- ◆ Irregular pupil—posterior synechiae
- ◆ Secondary glaucoma
- ◆ Secondary cataract
- ◆ Orbital pseudotumor
- ◆ Neuro-ophthalmologic
  - ◦ Visual field defects
  - ◦ Cranial nerve palsies
  - ◦ Optic neuropathy

Systemic Features

◆ Pulmonary
  ◦ Hilar lymphadenopathy
  ◦ Pulmonary infiltrates
  ◦ Pulmonary fibrosis
  ◦ Abnormal pulmonary function tests
◆ Neurologic
  ◦ Cranial nerve palsies
    ◆ Optic neuropathy
    ◆ Oculomotor nerve palsies
    ◆ Facial nerve palsy
    ◆ Acoustic nerve palsy
  ◦ Meningitis—usually chronic
  ◦ Hydrocephalus
  ◦ Cerebral granulomas with focal deficits
  ◦ Seizures
  ◦ Hypothalamic/pituitary dysfunction—granulomatous infiltration
  ◦ Cerebellar dysfunction
  ◦ Peripheral neuropathy
  ◦ Psychiatric disturbance
◆ Musculoskeletal
  ◦ Arthritis—acute or chronic
  ◦ Myositis
  ◦ Myopathies
  ◦ Bone cysts
◆ Skin
  ◦ Erythema nodosum
  ◦ Lupus pernio
  ◦ Skin nodules
  ◦ Rash
◆ Cardiac
  ◦ Pericarditis
  ◦ Cardiomyopathy
  ◦ Cardiac arrhythmias
◆ General
  ◦ Lymphadenopathy
  ◦ Hepatosplenomegaly
  ◦ Fever
  ◦ Anergy
  ◦ Hypercalcemia
  ◦ Hypercalcuria
  ◦ Abnormal liver enzymes
  ◦ Elevated serum angiotensin-converting enzyme (ACE) levels
  ◦ Elevated serum lysozyme
  ◦ Hypergammaglobulinemia
  ◦ Abnormal Kveim's skin test—rarely performed

33 Skin Disorders

◆ Albinism

Albinism refers to a group of genetic disorders of the melanocyte pigmentary system. They are characterized by hypopigmentation of skin, eyes, or both. Diagnosis of albinism is based on clinical findings. Tyrosinase activity can be evaluated by the hair bulb incubation test.

- ◆ Oculocutaneous albinism (OCA)—affects eyes, skin, and hair
  - ◦ Tyrosinase positive—some pigment is present; autosomal recessive inheritance; abnormal melanosome maturation. Affected individuals have white hair that turns yellowish with age, and pink irises that turn blue or hazel with age.
  - ◦ Tyrosinase negative—minimal pigment; autosomal recessive. The hair remains white, and the iris remains pink with age.
- ◆ Ocular albinism—Affected individuals have hypopigmentation of fundus and transillumination of iris. Skin may be slightly lighter than that of siblings. There is decreased number of melanocytes, normal melanosomes, and positive tyrosinase activity. Ocular albinism is transmitted as an X-linked recessive disorder. Males with the abnormal gene are always affected. Female carriers may have pigment mottling of fundus and partial iris transillumination.
- ◆ Other genetic variants are known to occur.

Fundus Features

- ◆ Hypopigmented fundus—"blond" fundus (**Figs. 33.1 and 33.2**)
- ◆ Visible choroidal vasculature—through hypopigmented retinal pigment epithelium (RPE) and choroid (**Fig. 33.3**)
- ◆ Foveal hypoplasia—abnormal foveal light reflex with absence of foveal pit
- ◆ Abnormal macular vasculature